Planning for Life
Involving adults with learning disabilities in service planning

T0187647

Can social care practitioners effectively involve people with learning disabilities in planning their services? Does user involvement for people with learning disabilities really benefit anyone?

Policy and practice guidelines for working with people with learning disabilities state that users and carers must be consulted in the provision of services. However, whether this is useful or effective in practice has not yet been adequately considered.

This book traces the development of services for people with disabilities and discusses how much things have really changed for today's 'service users' since the days of asylums. It also assesses whether the policy of involvement, such as that outlined in Valuing People, is achievable in practice or simply places unrealistic burdens on professionals and service users.

Based on findings from original research and interviews, the author argues that involving people with learning disabilities in service planning is difficult to achieve successfully and is currently, to a large extent, tokenistic. This area of challenging practice and emotive debate is brought to life by the voices of service providers, carers and the service users themselves, and illustrates the realities of working with people with learning disabilities.

Planning for Life will be valuable and informative for students of social work, social care and social policy, and will be enlightening reading for those working with adults with learning disabilities, in policy and in practice.

Liam Concannon is Lecturer in Social Policy and Social Work at Brunel University. He has experience of working with people with learning disabilities and currently teaches modules on mental health and learning disabilities in social work practice.

'Finally the head-nurse was sent for who seemed very kind and nice, and Dona went away with her very quietly and without a word as to whether we were coming too. She behaved so well throughout the whole proceeding, and I felt very much saying goodbye to the poor dear, leaving her amongst utter strangers and in a place not in the least suited to her. She also broke down just at the end. I wished I could have stayed longer with her at the end, but I felt very upset. After going round the Asylum, we went to a little restaurant and had some tea, and then left by train.'

A Young Woman's Diary from 1901

Planning for Life

Involving adults with learning disabilities in service planning

Liam Concannon

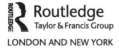
Routledge
Taylor & Francis Group

LONDON AND NEW YORK

First published in 2005 by Routledge
2 Park Square, Milton Park, Abingdon, Oxon OX14 4RN

Simultaneously published in the USA and Canada
by Routledge
711 Third Avenue, New York, NY 10017

Routledge is an imprint of the Taylor & Francis Group

© 2005 Liam Concannon

Typeset in 10/12 Sabon by J&L Composition, Filey, North Yorkshire

British Library Cataloguing in Publication Data
A catalogue record for this book is available from the British
Library

Library of Congress Cataloging in Publication Data
A catalogue record has been requested

ISBN 978-0-415-35156-0 (hbk)
ISBN 978-0-415-35157-7 (pbk)

Contents

Acknowledgements

There are many people I wish to thank for helping to make this study possible. First, my thanks go to the individuals and groups who took part in the interviews and group discussions which form the very heart of this research. For some, talking about their personal experiences proved to be difficult, and I thank them for sharing their ideas and speaking about their lives. Thanks also to the individuals who put me in touch with other groups and people.

A very special thanks goes to Sally Sainsbury at the London School of Economics. I thank her for her insight and support throughout, her inspiring enthusiasm and time. Thanks also to Professor David Denney at Royal Holloway, University of London and Professor Eric Sainsbury.

Lastly, Philip Maddock without whose encouragement this work would not have been completed.

Preface

Policies for people with learning disabilities, as in the case with other groups of service users, have increasingly emphasised the importance of their involvement in the planning of their own services, and at a more general level in the development of their local authority community care plan and commissioning strategies. The study on which this book is based seeks to begin to explore some of the difficulties that may arise in attempting to implement such a policy through a case study of practices in one inner London borough. The project includes a number of important interrelated themes including: the complexities of communication, normalisation, the nature of choice, citizenship and free will, and asks does social policy reform provision or create unrealistic expectations and burdens for social service professionals and service users?

The book is essentially about communication and its impact on choice and social inclusion. Focusing on communication between professionals and service users, their carers and advocates, the fieldwork investigates one council's strategic planning procedures in order to explore the relationship between service development and the preferences expressed by users. The findings are presented within a legislative framework, with particular interest paid to the government's White Papers *Modernising Social Services* and *Valuing People,* and the Best Value initiative. The project combines an historical account of policy development, and investigates social policies that have attempted to bring about change, while also exposing the contradictions within and between them. Because of this there are many challenges attached to this enterprise, and as a consequence the study is inevitably on a small scale and the answers it produces are tentative. Nevertheless it provides an indication of the nature and scale of the difficulties which social services will have to overcome if they are to make a reality of government policy in this area by engaging effectively with the personal experiences and lives of adults with learning disabilities and their carers.

Liam Concannon
November 2004

Introduction

An important medium through which local authorities seek to involve people with learning disabilities in service planning is consultation. Recently, the difficulties inherent in this process became clear to me when I attended a meeting set up by a social services department. The aim of the meeting was to consult people with learning disabilities, their families and carers about the services they received from a large independent sector provider organisation in the borough, which for reasons of confidentiality, will be referred to as Octa throughout this study. Octa had, for a number of years, relied on the social services department for funding in order to provide their services and pay staff. However, there was growing concern among senior managers and budget holders about the effect that the escalating costs of Octa's services were having on the learning disability budget. Because of an overspend the previous year, the learning disability section had been directed to find savings, and in light of this some services Octa offered, although of great value to the users and families, had simply become too expensive for the department, resulting in changes needing to be made and savings found. The professionals argued that a number of services provided by Octa had over the years become duplicated and gave the example of the outreach service. The managers said that both Octa and social services had outreach teams, which meant that not only was the department paying for its own in-house staff, but it was also funding Octa to carry out the same work often with the same service users.

Some parents and carers attending the meeting had a long involvement with Octa, and were understandably defensive and angry with the senior managers about the proposed changes. The families were out to 'fight' to keep hold of what they saw as *their* services. Most, however, were less than skilled when it came to debating their point, and it was not long before the meeting descended into a heated argument on the part of the parents and carers, with threats to involve the local newspaper and the local MP. Many of the service users present were confused and uninformed. Most at best could not articulate an argument, and at worst had no identifiable means of communication with anyone. As I looked around the room I noticed one man who sat rocking in his chair with his eyes fixed on the ceiling continually and rapidly tapping his fingers on the side of his nose, while another young woman wandered around the room picking up objects and smelling them. As she walked around she made a monotone noise, a kind of 'mmmm' sound. It was unclear why she had been brought along to the consultation meeting, and how she was expected to make any kind of contribution to the decisions about the future of services being discussed. When the service users were asked for their thoughts regarding the services that they wanted, one woman in a sing-song voice replied, 'I like Julie, I like Monday club,' and then burst into laughter. Another simply repeated, 'la la la la shooopink, shooopink', several times over. Looking around I found myself asking the fundamental question: *How is it possible to involve people with learning disabilities in service planning?* And more to the point, with the communication and cognitive difficulties experienced by many of these people: *Is it actually possible for them to make valid choices?* I questioned why many of these people had been brought along, people who clearly could not articulate their needs and choices. Given the appalling, and often downright cruel, history of treatment towards people with learning disabilities, I was also curious to know why this group of people continued to be treated as a 'Cinderella' service even after the publication of many promising pieces of legislation and social policy designed to improve their lives? It seemed important to explore systematically the obstacles to their serious incorporation into the consultation process.

Any attempt to research the views of people with learning disabilities is likely to be fraught with problems. Yet in recent years, involving users in service planning has been given a high profile by the government. The recently published White Paper[1] *Modernising Social Services,* discusses the 1998 Annual Report of the Joint Reviews stating that:

> . . . in most cases councils are not reviewed unless required by law. The finding is underpinned by the user and carer's experience. Many report that they have not been asked how things are going. Many users and carers have valuable knowledge about services, but many councils are not asking them to share this knowledge.[2]

Consulting people with learning disabilities about the services they receive is a relatively new concept. One function it has, in theory at least, is as a way of asking the user about *choice.* Asking people with learning disabilities about their wishes and choices helps to identify both their wants and needs, and should enable professionals to find ways for services to best meet those needs.

Although examining the views of people with learning disabilities is a growing area for research, it is still very much in its infancy. One of the biggest problems this project found was linking the current literature about choice and social inclusion to the everyday experiences of people with learning disabilities. A substantial literature exists on how to carry out social research in general terms, but there are few examples of practical methodologies that can be used when researching the views of people with communication and cognitive difficulties. No single method would be satisfactory for this type of research largely because of problems concerning understanding. For this reason it was a case of 'mixing and matching' from the main body of literature available on social research methods, communication skills, and previous disability research. The approach to the fieldwork was open and as flexible as possible. Previous studies concerning the lives of people with learning disabilities have tended to look at what the professionals have had to say about consulting users and involving them in decisions. The fieldwork carried out for this study broke new ground because it brought together the thoughts and experiences of the users, professionals, parents and carers regarding current practice and policies in order to compare and contrast these views. However, ultimately only interview material from those people with learning disabilities who could understand what the research sought, and who could make themselves understood, could be included. Observation was used; not only to deepen an appreciation of the feelings and views of those interviewed, but also to include those whose communication and cognitive problems excluded them from the interview process.

This work investigates the process of involving people with learning disabilities in service planning. It traces the history of services to this group, exploring aspects of policy past and present that have influenced and shaped the lives of these people from the rise of eugenics, to the impact of the normalisation and ordinary life discourse. Finally, it will investigate the reality of care in the community from the Thatcherite ideology of the early 1980s through to New Labour and the Blair administration.

NOTES

1 Department of Health, *Modernising Social Services, Promoting Independence, Improving Protection, Raising Standards*, Cm. 4169 (London: HMSO, 1998), p. 15.
2 Joint Reviews of Social Services are carried out by the Social Services Inspectorate (SSI) and the Audit Commission. They combine the service expertise of the SSI with the Audit Commission's understanding of value for money and effectiveness. The reviews investigate the performance of each authority across the whole of its social services responsibilities, and produce a published report. The Joint Reviews cover 20 authorities each year, and have so far published reports on 27 of the 150 councils responsible for social services in England.

1 The historical and social context of care to people with learning disabilities

> . . . the best of our men with the best of our women as often as possible, and the inferior men with the inferior women as seldom as possible, bringing up only the offspring of the best . . . the children of the inferior Guardians, and any others, will be quietly and secretly disposed of.[3]

The quote above could easily be taken from the policies of the Nazi Party during the Second World War. In fact it comes from a much earlier era, that of classical Greece, and demonstrates the extent to which the concept of eugenics has been engrained in the human psyche throughout history. The passage is from *The Republic*, a work in which Plato outlines a programme of eugenics, and in a similar manner, the Socratic emphasis was on knowledge and reason with the aim of establishing a hierarchy based on intellectual capacity and reason. Aristotle developed the theme of eugenics in much the same style, outlining methods for regulating the marriages of those who it was expected would produce the best quality offspring. Expectant mothers of good offspring were to be taken care of during pregnancy while at the other extreme, he advocates in favour of a 'law that no cripple child shall be reared'.[4] There are many interesting facets to Plato's scheme of selective breeding, but perhaps one of the most significant is the suggestion that it would need to be carried out in secret. This was because he expected there would be a negative reaction towards the practice.[5] It must be carried out in the dark because of sentiment in families and the care that parents have towards their children, and this despite the widespread practice of exposing infants in classical Greece.

In *De Anima*, Aristotle argues that there is a strong association between reason, goodness and humanness and he defines the soul under three headings: (1) the *nutritive soul*, common to all living organisms which is concerned with basic self-nurturing, (2) the *sensitive soul*, characterised by the ability to perceive through sight and sounds and is common to both man and animals, and (3) the *rational soul*, characterised by the capacity for cognition.[6] What Aristotle presents here is an order to the soul by suggesting a natural hierarchy that differentiates man from animals.[7] As the classical period drew to a close three central themes emerge from the history which defines 'the idiot': (1) *an association with animals*, (2) *as objects of amusement, and* (3) *inherently inferior*. It was not until a much later period, with the advent of Christianity, that attitudes towards 'the idiot' saw a significant change brought about through Christian theology. From Christianity came the doctrines of compassion, universal love, charity and grace, and Christians were urged by theologians: 'Now we exhort you, brethren . . . comfort the feeble-minded . . . be patient with all men' (1 Thessalonians 5:14). For the most part it was, and continues to be, such doctrines that have had the most significant impact on attitudes and social responses towards people with learning disabilities throughout history. It is interesting that during the medieval period grace became the most significant of these doctrines, because of the belief that man would be saved by the *Grace of God* and not his own reason. A further Christian doctrine, that of *original sin*, carried with it an unexpected status of equality for 'the idiot'.[8] Theologians argued original sin was so great a turning away from God by *all* of mankind, that any inequality of status between individuals on earth was insignificant in the eyes of God.[9] One of the foremost contributors to the Church's discourse on Grace and the Fall from God was St Augustine (AD 354–430). Augustine in his work *Anti-Pelagian*[10] offers some insight into the life of 'an idiot' during this period. Most importantly in this work it becomes clear how those deemed 'idiots' first became labelled as *'the holy innocents'*. Augustine, discussing original sin and connecting his argument to children, suggests that children are baptised as a means of cleansing them from original sin, not because they have sinned. Augustine observes that because children cannot 'reason' their 'folly' cannot be considered sins for which they are responsible. Hence they are considered the 'holy innocents' and he compares the folly of children with that of the 'monriones' noting:

> '. . . by their own will . . . infants could never commit an offence, the habit of calling *innocent*? Does not their great weakness of mind and body, their great ignorance of things . . . the absence in them of all perception and impression of law, either natural or written, the complete want of reason to impel them in either direction, – proclaim and demonstrate the point before us.[11]

This position argues that the holy innocents lack the capacity to knowingly sin, and here begins the association between children and those deemed 'idiots', and for some it is an association and imagery that has continued throughout history to the present day. Yet these ideas have often been associated with people with learning disabilities to justify great cruelty. Some of the reforming ideas which began to develop in the early 19th century, were to merge before the end of the century through the eugenics movement associated with Darwinian biology, with which many progressive thinkers, especially in the field of social policy, were involved. But progressives in

Britain ultimately failed to convince legislators of the necessity for forcible sterilisation in 1913 (see p. 35). It was in Nazi Germany that their ideas were to find their most complete practical expression. There eugenicists were able to move from a programme of forcible sterilisation of people with learning disabilities, to one of elimination. In Britain, from the 1930s ideas began to change direction, and this, together with the Nazi sterilisation and elimination policies, ensured that from the end of the Second World War, eugenics could not be spoken of in polite society. That new British direction culminated in current policies based on ideas about choices and rights. Yet alongside these policies new developments have emerged which suggest a revival of eugenics in a new guise.

Let us now consider how the doctrine of grace could be used to ends so widely distant from those of its originators. In 1530, Paracelsus[12] attempted to re-examine the concept of the doctrine of Grace by investigating the nature of knowledge.[13] Paracelsus concluded that in the eyes of God all men were equal. He argued 'the fool' was equal to the common man, seeing the true soul as trapped within the fool's animal body, but also warns man about growing arrogant within the boundaries of his animal reason:

> . . . and know ye also withal that the fools reveal greater judgement, more shrewdness, more wisdom than the wise. Because wisdom comes from the true man, who does not die, and it does not come from the animal body, yet through the animal body it shows itself and is revealed . . . thus the animal reason that is with us, which we regard as great and intelligent, and of which we think highly, and through which we want to accomplish much, stands in relation to the reason which the true man has [the inner reason of the soul] as such fools are regarded in relation to us. That is we scorn them because they do not control their reason.[14]

Ultimately, however, it was the state, drawing on this idea of the lack of responsibility of the innocents, not the Church, that attempted to determine the status of the 'idiot'; for example, with regard to the right of property. At the beginning of the 14th century laws of competence were passed for the control of those called 'idiots', both in England and Europe. In England laws concerned themselves with the *guardianship* of 'the idiot' and attitudes towards 'idiots' changed; no longer seeing them as a source of amusement, the lawmakers now moved to a position whereby 'the idiot' needed to be controlled. Thus from the Renaissance era emerged the dual themes of *control* and *paternalism*. During the 16th and 17th centuries, the law increasingly recognised a need to control 'idiots' for their own good, offering terms of reference such as *identification* and *definition*. One of the earliest definitions recorded during this era came from the writing of Sir Anthony Fitzherbert who in 1534 published *New Natura Brevium* classifying 'the idiot' as 'such a person who cannot account or number twenty pence, nor can tell who was his father or mother'.[15] During the early 1700s, the laws had been formulated sufficiently to produce the *Law Relating to Natural Fools and Mad Folk*, published by John Brydall, and shortly after this moves towards incarceration and confinement came swiftly into being. Workhouses, originating in the Tudor Poor Laws, became the mainstay of institutional care for any of the poor who were categorised as 'idiots'.

With the dawning of the *Age of Reason*, once again came a shift in attitudes, this time moving away from Christian doctrines to 'educating the idiot'. For 'the idiot', the Age of Reason would turn out to be one of the most productive and positive periods in history with characters like Tuke and Pinel emerging to take centre-stage. It must be remembered however, that for the most part the 'idiot' and the 'mad' continued to be treated as indistinguishable (see pp. 35–6). Philippe Pinel (1745–1826) was a French physician who pioneered the humane treatment of 'the idiot'. In 1792, Pinel became the chief physician at Bicêtre, the Paris asylum for men, where many inmates had been restrained for 30 or 40 years. Pinel rejected the long-held and popular beliefs about 'the idiot' and the 'mad' as individuals who were *demonically possessed*. He did away with common treatments such as bleeding, purging, and blistering instead favouring therapies that included close friendly contact with the patient.[16] 'Idiots' and 'the mad' were often believed to be devoid of human feeling which had resulted in their treatment being indifferent, brutal and cruel. Pinel scandalised his fellow physicians by reversing these practices, removing the chains from inmates at Bicêtre. He believed that 'lunacy' was the result of some form of bodily disease, and his method and treatment were simple in that he replaced cruelty with kindness, taking the inmates out of their dungeons and giving them sunny rooms, with the liberty to walk around pleasant grounds. Pinel developed his own exercises for mental distress based on observation and reason. What was striking and unique about Pinel's work during this period of history was the compassion he demonstrated. When asked by the revolutionary Couthon 'Are you mad yourself to unchain such beasts?', Pinel replied, 'Citizen, I am convinced that these madmen are so intractable only because they have been deprived of air and liberty.'[17] During the late 1700s, while Pinel was developing his work in France, a similar approach was being adopted by Samuel Tuke (1784–1857) in York, England.[18] There is no evidence to suggest that these two knew each other or ever met, each worked independently but the results they arrived at, and their methods, were strikingly similar. Tuke's approach to his work was theological, based on the Quaker belief in the Inner Light.[19] He opened a house at York that became known as The Retreat. It is interesting to note that although The Retreat was at one of the great ecclesiastical centres of England, no encouragement for the compassionate work of Tuke came from either the Archbishop of York or any of his clergy, perhaps a tribute to the power and influence of the Governors of the York Asylum.[20] Indeed the opposite was true. Tuke's ideas, like those of grace and holy innocence, were subject to effective assault from the new and increasingly powerful reforming Methodist movement. The ideas generated by John Wesley, founder of the Methodist movement, had a powerful impact on people's ideas, and these in relation to people deemed 'idiots' are instructive. Speaking of 'lunatics', he sees the source of their behaviour in demonic possession. It was the theological position that continued to have a damning influence and control over people's thinking towards 'the idiot'. Consider the following approach adopted by John Wesley where he speaks about 'the lunatic' as being demonically possessed. Wesley:

> insisted on the authority of the Old Testament, that bodily diseases are sometimes caused by devils, and, upon the authority of the New Testament, that the gods of the heathen are demons; he believed that dreams, while in some cases caused by bodily conditions and passions, are shown by Scripture to be also caused by occult powers of evil; he cites a physician to prove that "most lunatics are really demoniacs." In his great sermon Evil Angels, he dwells upon this point especially; resists the idea that "possession" may be epilepsy, even though ordinary symptoms of epilepsy be present; protests against giving up to infidels such proofs of an invisible world as are to be found in diabolic possession; and evidently believes that some who have been made hysterical by his own preaching are possessed of Satan.[21]

The growth of early institutions was rapid, however, attitudes towards the care of 'idiots' began to shift once more in both Europe and Britain. This was due to a new generation of professionals who were determined to instil religious and moral values into the minds of their patients. For British evangelicals the object was saving souls. However, at a time of burgeoning interest in social problems a multiplicity of ideas began to develop in relation to the treatment of 'idiots', any one of which had the possibilities of political influence.

At the same time in Britain no state laws existed that specifically recognised 'the idiot' as a separate category needing specific care. Laws governing them emanated from more general legislation such as the Poor Law Act (1844) and the Lunatic Asylum Act (1853). Both laws made institutional provision for those regarded as 'idiots'.

By 1875 the Committee for Considering the Best Means of Making Satisfactory Provision for Idiots, Imbeciles and Harmless Lunatics had been established and included among its members Tuke, J. Langdon Down and W. W. Ireland. These men were out to change the social order, arguing, for example, that asylums and workhouses were not appropriate places for the care of this group of people, but called for special provision to be made for them.[22] The committee wanted the Metropolitan Poor Act of 1867 extended to include special measures aimed at

> elevating them to the highest level of which their organisation admits, curing them of their offensive habits, affording them some positive happiness, and shielding them from unkind and irritating treatment.[23]

Further, it recommended establishing new 'idiot' asylums which Tuke supported suggesting that 'schools' of up to 500 could be set up to cater to the needs of those who 'having been trained ... to a certain point' had reached a stage 'beyond which it is impossible to train them'.[24] The committee produced a report which contributed to the first piece of legislation to be introduced specifically for 'idiots': the Idiots Act 1886.[25] The Act was brief, only four pages long in total, and had no significant impact on services. Regardless, the eugenics movement was growing in support; its influences could be seen as 'unscientific do-gooders' were swept aside in favour of the 'voice of reason'.[26] Language also reflected this change with the word 'school' replaced by 'asylum', with 'the idiot' moving from needing protection from society to being a character from whom society needed to be protected. The growth of influence of scientific interest in the subject, out of which eugenics was to grow, is to be found in the work of two of Tuke's contemporaries and initially that interest focused on classification.

EARLY CLASSIFICATION

J. Langdon Down (1828–96) is probably the most famous name associated with the early classification of people with learning disabilities. A philanthropist and physician Langdon Down was superintendent of Earlswood Asylum in Surrey from 1858 to 1868. He classified systems that highlighted differing grades of 'idiot', based primarily on ethnicity, and did this by carrying out post-mortems on former patients as a method for identifying a range of ethnic groupings. Langdon Down also used the post-mortems as a means for examining the cranial capacity investigating anatomical differences. His findings were published in 1887 and included the 'Mongoloid' term that came to bear his name 'Down's Syndrome'.[27] Another prominent figure associated with early classification was William Wotherspoon Ireland (1832–1909). Ireland published a comprehensive medical text on 'the idiot' in 1887. He had trained as a physician and in 1869 was appointed the first superintendent of the Scottish National Institute at Larbert. Ireland agreed with Langdon Down's system of classification, adding new dimensions such as the proposed classification based mainly on physical characteristics. Langdon Down gave little consideration to applying a psychological approach to his patients, while Ireland in a similar manner gave little consideration to psychiatric matters. The main aim and purpose of classification at this point in history was to identify those individuals who could benefit from social training and who could be educated away from their 'dirty habits'. However, eugenics as an aspect of science was beginning to be investigated seriously.

THE RISE OF EUGENICS

> Early [in the 20th] century, mentally handicapped people were considered a eugenic threat and large numbers of relatively mildly handicapped people were placed in institutions where the sexes were segregated. Today, many attempts to establish new community residential services for mentally handicapped people are met by objections, often based on erroneous notions of 'danger' to local people, children, pets, property or property values.[28]

Sir Francis Galton (1822–1911) is considered to be the founder of the science of eugenics. He coined the term eugenics in 1883 taking it from the Greek meaning 'good-born'. The theory was based on Charles Darwin's principle of natural selection and Galton applied it to society. An English anthropologist, Galton collected statistics on the physical characteristics of large numbers of people, and is most commonly remembered for his work on devising a method of identification by fingerprinting. Galton began his work on eugenics around 1865 by measuring the human faculties, tracing similarities and differences in families through successive generations. These early studies led him to formulate what he termed 'ancestral law' and in 1869 he published *Hereditary Genius: An Inquiry into Its Laws and Consequences.*[29] This work set out to prove there existed a *law of distribution of ability* in families. His work inferred that if eminent people mated with eminent people, the process would produce eminent people. His contemporary critics, however, argued that the flaw in Galton's theory was that by creating only eminent people, the race as a whole would become unbalanced resulting in an unworkable society coming into existence.

According to his theory the genetic quality of the human race can be improved and Galton defined his science of eugenics as 'the science of improvement of the human race germ plasma through better breeding'.[30] The science proposed two distinct areas, those of *heredity* and the *environmental*, and Galton believed that heredity was by far the more important of the two. The basis for his theory began with simple observations made about the breeding of racehorses. Horses were bred for strength and so Galton argued men could be bred in the same way and with the same aim. From the time eugenics began to find support at the end of the 19th century, it held to two philosophical convictions:

- a growth in the belief that the human species could be perfected;
- a belief that science was the most dependable form of knowledge.[31]

Eugenicists suggested the key to creating a better society was the 'proper breeding of good stock' stressing that proper breeding was the only means by which the human condition is controlled and improved. Two further characteristics emerged from the eugenics movement during this period: the first was the need to concentrate on *increasing* the breeding of 'fit' individuals, and the second emphasised the need to *restrict* the breeding of the 'unfit'. From its earliest days the movement aligned good breeding with white Anglo-Saxon superiority, but this was a superiority which had to be worked at to be sustained. Eugenics was to have a wide-ranging and long-lasting influence on society about those who were 'different'.

Impact of eugenics: the segregation of 'the idiot'

Limited reference to the care of 'the idiot' had been introduced in the 1886 Idiots Act, but the later Lunacy Act of 1890 was felt to be a retrogressive step, in that it did not make a distinction between the needs of people with a mental illness and those deemed 'idiots'. It was not until the much later Mental Deficiency Act of 1913, that the foundation for some form of need for formal establishment of separate service provision was recognised. What the 1913 Act sought to achieve was care *out* of the community, and it aimed to classify those people deemed 'mentally ill' and segregate them from the *'mentally subnormal'*. For the 'subnormal', emphasis began to be placed on their *active* care with attempts made to train them.

Policy makers from the mid-19th century until the early part of the 20th century were responsible for a considerable increase in the number and size of mental subnormality hospitals. It was a commonly held belief that such institutions were beneficial places where people could receive appropriate care. Here the 'mentally subnormal' could be identified, controlled and monitored. The following allows a glimpse into the regime of life inside one of these institutions during the mid-19th century.

> The modern institution is generally a large one, preferably built on a colony plan, takes defectives of all grades and all ages. All, of course, are probably classified according to their mental capacity and age . . . An institution which takes all types and ages is economical because the high grade patients do the work and make everything necessary, not only for themselves, but also for the lower grade. In an institution taking only lower grades, the whole of the work has to be done by paid staff; in one taking only high grades the output of work is greater than is required for the institution itself and there is difficulty in disposing of it. In all-grade institutions . . . the high grade patients are skilled

workmen of the colony, those who do all the higher processes of man-
ufacture, those on whom there is a considerable measure of responsibility; the medium grade patients are the labourers, . . . the rest of the
lower grade patients fetch and carry or do simple work . . .[32]

From the 1860s there had been a growing demand from society for greater
segregation of the 'mentally subnormal'. One of the popular reasons of the
day then offered was to safeguard the interests of society and stop any form
of *contamination* by association taking place. Anyone deemed 'mad' or
'subnormal' was a danger to society and, therefore, the responsible answer
to the problem was to remove them from the community. The asylums were
run along colony principles and were closely regulated controlled communities. Goffman (1968)[33] describes them as 'total institutions', Foucault
(1967)[34] as 'structures of confinement', and Scull (1979)[35] as 'museums of
madness', places that played a major part in the social construction of mental deficiency, acting as dumping-grounds for society's undesirables. An
example of how this operated is given in the case of the woman, taken to
an institution as a moral defective, because she gave birth to an illegitimate
child with no means of providing for the child except through poor relief.
A letter from this period written by the Lancashire and Cheshire Society for
the Care of the Feeble Minded declared:

> The weaker the intellect the greater appears to be the strength of the
> reproduction facilities. It is as though when the higher faculties have
> dwindled, the lower, or merely animal, take command.[36]

Asylums needed to be strictly controlled and regulated environments especially taking into account the scale and size of many of these institutions.
They were run in a similar way to the workhouses of the time but with one
main distinction, asylums were committed to training their inmates. It is
difficult with the current climate of care in the community, and the anti-
institution movement, to understand the optimism on which the asylum of
the mid-19th century was founded:

> Buildings that now fill us with despair were seen as model environ-
> ments full of promise in which could occur the creation of economi-
> cally independent and morally competent individuals by a
> combination of moral training and task-centred learning in an envi-
> ronment that emphasised health, nutrition, exercise and the creation
> of habits of discipline.[37]

This optimistic expectation of the era was clearly demonstrated in the
notion that 'the subnormal' could be trained and educated and to an extent
'normalised'. The institution's teaching regime held out the hope that people could develop skills of self-care. They were taught to eat properly, dress

and undress themselves, keep themselves clean and tidy and where possible become articulate. With *high grades* the eventual goal was to enable them to read and write. The following are extracts taken from the Western Counties Asylums (WCA) Annual Report 1902, highlighting what the institutions felt they were achieving:

> O.P. a boy of twelve when admitted was very backward in all branches of learning and could not use a pencil . . . by careful and continuous training . . . he is now able to write fairly in a copy book and to do sums of long division.'
>
> L.F. This girl came to us from a home for feeble-minded girls and could neither read nor write. She can now read easy tales and write so well that her friends are delighted with the letters she sends home to them. She has moreover become quite a good housemaid.[38]

Of course for most 'subnormals' the experience was somewhat different. In 1855, one of the largest asylums to be built in Britain was opened at Earlswood, Surrey. The asylum could accommodate up to 500 patients and was unique for the period, because it was one of the first asylums specifically for 'the mentally subnormal'. Britain, unlike most other countries, made a distinct separation between 'the mentally subnormal' and those with 'a mental illness'. Earlswood's programme of education was innovatory and individuals, essentially from wealthy families, were sent there from all over the country and, in some cases, the world.[39] The experience of putting someone away in an institution was a difficult and emotional process, which often proved to be just as upsetting for family members as it was for the individual. Diaries found recently, written at the turn of the 20th century, recount one such story of a woman in 1901, who recalls her journey to England from India with her Aunt Louie and Aunt Dona; the latter was an 'incurable'. They came by boat from India where Dona had lived with her family since she was born. Their journey was to end at Earlswood Asylum. At the time of writing the diaries the woman was 21 years old and Dona 40. The passage demonstrates the absolute powerlessness and hopelessness Dona had over her own circumstances and her future life:

'A Young Woman's Diary from 1901.'[40]

Thursday 21 March 1901

Aunt Louie, Dona and I left by the Bombay mail for Bombay . . . It was very sad leaving the old place after its being Dona and my home for so many years, and where we have had troubles as well as happy days.

Saturday 13 April 1901

We got to Gravesend at 6 o'clock in the morning and at 8 we arrived in the docks. The Martins came at the appointed time. Had the papers signed by the ship's Doctor about Dona . . . I can still hardly realise that I am actually in England.

Saturday 27 April 1901

I finished all Dona's packing in the morning. Dona was a little cross about being sent to school, which ended in a little cry, doing her ever so much good, as she got more composed after that. We had early lunch, then started in a cab for Victoria, taking three quarters of an hour to drive there, but the way did not seem long, as there are so many interesting places and things to be seen en route. We got to Victoria in due time, and Dona and I sat in the ladies waiting room while Percy went to meet the Martins on another platform. After a wait of about half an hour at Victoria we all got onto the train for Earlswood arriving there at quarter past two, then walked to the Asylum which is a beautiful big place with grounds laid out like a park. We had to wait in an audience room 'till the Doctor came; he asked Dona a good many questions, which she answered very well, and then we were questioned as to a good many things. Finally the head-nurse was sent for who seemed very kind and nice, and Dona went away with her very quietly and without a word as to whether we were coming too. She behaved so well throughout the whole proceeding, and I felt very much saying goodbye to the poor dear, leaving her amongst utter strangers and in a place not in the least suited to her. She also broke down just at the end. I wished I could have stayed longer with her at the end, but I felt very upset. After going round the Asylum, we went to a little restaurant and had some tea, and then left by train again, the Martins getting off at Clapham Junction, and we going on to Victoria, and then by underground to Hampstead. I was glad to get once more to my room to give way to my pent up feelings.

Wednesday 7 August 1901

. . . We had lunch early as I was going down to Earlswood to see Dona, and Percy had some business in town. So we went together as far as Victoria, and parted there. Dona was looking very well but she still says that she does not like staying there and she would like to come home again. I took her out to tea which she enjoyed, then on her return to the Asylum, we sat in the grounds and heard the band play-ing 'Patience', so it seemed quite familiar. Got home later than usual as the trains were late.

Wednesday 27 November 1901

Had an early lunch, then started for Victoria, met Aunt Louie there, and we both went to Earlswood to see Dona. We found her looking very well, but she was so silent, and seemed so sad, almost the only thing she said of her own accord was that she would like to go home. I think she must be lonely there, having to be kept so much apart from the others, and it is very pitiful when she asks to come home. I do feel so much for the poor dear soul. I only wish we were nearer to get to see her oftener.

Dona died in 1932 aged 72 years and Earlswood as an asylum finally closed its doors in March 1997.

THE ROYAL COMMISSION OF 1904–8: PATERNALISM AND CONTROL

During the early part of the 20th century there was a growing dissatisfac-tion from the public about the degeneration of society. It was largely due to such concern that the *Royal Commission on the Care and Control of the Feeble-Minded* was set up in 1904.[41] The commission sat for four years investigating provisions for 'mental incurables' and went as far as visiting the United States to look at services in that country. The result was that the commission produced the *Report and Minutes of Evidence.*[42] What was uniquely interesting about the report was that it captures a period of tran-sition in British history where society moves from a time that is humane and paternalistic to one of suppression and control. The report portrays the shift from moralism and science to the development of a hardcore eugenic thinking with tensions between paternalism and control. The importance of control can be seen running throughout the report and from the beginning the commission was charged with considering:

> . . . existing methods of dealing with idiots and epileptics and with imbecile, feeble-minded or defective persons . . . in view of such hard-ship or danger resulting to such persons and the community from insufficient provision for their care, training and control.[43]

Ultimately the report, despite its harsh tones, reflected the principles of paternalism over control suggesting that the 'mentally defective' 'should be afforded by the state such special protection as may be suited to their needs'.[44] Moreover, though under pressure from eugenicists, the commission considered, but rejected, sterilisation, arguing that the protection and well-being of 'defectives', not the purification of the race, should provide the main grounds for action. This is the first occasion in history when it was recognised that the needs of people with learning disabilities were going to be met by the state, which, as noted by the commission, was new to English law.

THE MENTAL DEFICIENCY ACT 1913

Influenced by the ideas developing in the field of eugenics, the Mental Deficiency Act 1913 was introduced with the principal aim of committing 'mental defectives' to a life away from the community in large isolated and rural institutions. One of the many problems with the 1913 Act was the way in which it used the term 'mental deficiency'. The definition given spanned a large and loose range of meanings from 'mental incurables' and 'feeble-minded idiots', to 'moral imbeciles' and individuals accused of loose morals. As a consequence it was often the case that the people committed to an asylum under the 1913 Act, were guilty of little more than a one-off anti-social act. A Board of Control was set up as a result of the Act and had the task of admitting and discharging patients to and from institutions, and the board also held the responsibility for care of the patients once committed.

By 1913 asylums had undergone a substantial transformation becoming places where less emphasis was placed on the improvement of inmates, who were increasingly pooled together resulting in a loss of personal identity, and educational development with individuality giving way to a mass organisation of daily life. The 1913 Act did, however, recognise and make some provision for those individuals who neither were suited to life in an institution nor required statutory guardianship. It directed local authorities to set up an administrative structure to cater to the needs of those who remained in the community which, when established, became known as the *Mental Deficiency Committee* (1926). The Board of Control argued against care in the community suggesting it was unsatisfactory compared with the care an individual could receive in one of the large institutions. The examples presented in the WCA Report 1902 of O.P., a boy of 12, and L.F. a 'feeble-minded' girl, who were taught to read, write and do sums are good illustrations of the board's reasons for their stance in favour of institutional care.

THE CASE FOR AND AGAINST THE 'INTELLIGENCE QUOTIENT'

Despite the certainty of objectives among eugenicists there remained considerable uncertainty regarding the definition and classification of those regarded as 'idiots'. Historically, the *'idiot'* suffered from an incurable congenital condition, whereas it was suggested, the *'lunatic'* had only a temporary loss of reason. The *essence* of 'the idiot', therefore, was a lack of development, whereas 'the mad' were suffering from a temporary imbalance but were still capable of some effective and logical thinking. The language used in early legislation, such as with the Mental Deficiency Act 1913, reflected how much of a social, rather than a medical, problem these people were with descriptions such as 'idiot', 'imbecile', 'feeble-minded' and 'moral defective'.

There had been a search to find a method of applying scientific principles to the classification of 'mental defectives' and one that would explain the arrested development of the mind. In 1908 Binet and Simon were the first to publish the results of a series of tests examining *'Intelligence Quotient'*. These tests explored the notion of mental age in relation to chronological age. Binet and Simon argued that mental ability was part of an individual's basic psychological make-up and functioning that could not be changed over time. The implications of this suggested intellectual ability are 'fixed' at birth and no amount of learning or social change could alter this. Their opinions were embraced by the medical profession and welcomed most notably by members of the eugenics society. One of the most ardent proponents in favour of segregating mental defectives was Tredgold, a leading specialist in 'mental deficiency' and an exponent of eugenics, who in 1909 suggested it was the social inefficiency of the 'defectives', regardless of IQ, that should be the means by which they were classified. Tredgold's comments largely reflected the mood of many progressives of the day when he observed:

> . . . as soon as a nation reaches that stage of civilisation in which medical knowledge and humanitarian sentiment operate to prolong the existence of the unfit, then it becomes imperative upon that nation to devise such social laws as will ensure that those unfit do not propagate their kind.[45]

In the *Eugenics Review* (1909) Tredgold makes plain his case:

- In the first place the chief evil we have to prevent is undoubtedly that of propagation.
- Next, society must protect against such of these persons as either have definite criminal tendencies, or are of so facile a disposition that they readily commit crimes at the instigation of others.
- Lastly, even where these poor creatures are relatively harmless, we have to protect society from the burden due to their non-productiveness.[46]

Views like that of Tredgold were highly influential in ensuring the format that the Mental Deficiency Act 1913 would take. Objections from Parliament had arisen when in 1912 a Mental Deficiency Bill had been introduced. The Bill, based on very solid eugenic views, had included the prohibition of 'the mentally deficient' from marrying. Parliamentary opposition was such that the Bill was later withdrawn the same year only to be replaced by what many regarded as the much harsher 1913 Act. The prohibition of marriage was removed but replaced by a much greater emphasis on *keeping people* in institutions once they had been admitted. Institutions became convenient repositories for people who often did not require institutionalisation and who could have lived productive lives in the community. They were incarcerated solely because they were seen as social undesirables with a low IQ.

Because of the policy of incarceration, and to achieve economies of scale, the size of institutions grew, in some cases accommodating up to 2,000 patients. Tredgold had demanded large isolated colonies where the number of people involved grew steadily, increasing from 12,000 in 1920 to 100,000 in 1950. Tredgold offers his findings, summarised in Table 1, saying the figures are for those people under 'the various forms of care'.[47] However, he fails to make it clear whether they were incarcerated in asylums during these years.

THE MENTAL DEFICIENCY ACT 1927 AND THE WOOD COMMITTEE REPORT 1929

By 1927, a revised version of the Mental Deficiency Act was produced and when the Wood Committee Report was published in 1929, together they marked a significant turning-point in attitudes towards the mentally subnormal and their care. The emphasis yet again shifted, this time to care *outside* the institution. The Wood Committee had recommended that 'mental defectives' should come under the responsibility of the mental deficiency authorities, and with the reorganisation of local government

Table 1 Total number of defectives under the care and control of the Mental Deficiency Act

Year	Total number (rounded up)
1920	12,000
1926	37,000
1939	90,000
1950	100,000

Source: A. F. Tredgold, assisted by R. F. Tredgold, *A Textbook on Mental Deficiency (Amentia)* (London: Bailliére, 1952)

brought about by the Local Government Act 1929, this became possible. It was also around this period that a body of expertise began to be developed centred on the needs of 'the subnormal', with specialist training programmes for welfare officers, teachers and other professionals. There was a growing awareness of the value that remaining at home could offer to these people reflected in the passing of the Mental Treatment Act in 1930, which sought to further positive attitudes towards care outside the institution. However, in the United States of America the opposite approach had been slowly emerging with the rise in eugenic thinking becoming a powerful force for racial bias and suppression.

EUGENIC THINKING

The early eugenics movement and the United States of America

It was in the United States, not Nazi Germany, that the first large-scale sterilisation policy was implemented with more than 30,000 people, considered 'abnormal', sterilised in 29 states between 1907 and 1939. Most of these individuals were sterilised against their will and without an understanding of what was happening to them. The majority were incarcerated in institutions for 'subnormals' and the 'mentally ill' or in prisons, and the sterilisation programmes both in the United States and later in Germany were strongly influenced by eugenicist theories.[48]

In America eugenics found a powerful base becoming a forceful movement for overt racial bias that became reflected in the state and federal laws of the era. Eugenics suggested that one of the greatest threats to society was 'the reproduction of defectives by defectives', and for this reason many parents who had 'retarded' children sought, and were encouraged to seek, sterilisation for their child. These parents saw sterilisation, not as a choice but as a social duty and responsibility they had to take to safeguard their child. This was largely fuelled by the belief that both male and female 'defectives' had strong sexual inclinations to reproduce, coupled with poor personal control, thus making them a menace to society. The suggestion was that:

> the inhibitive nerve power is weakened, the lower nature is apt to assert itself. Though children in mind, they are often men and women in wickedness and vice.[49]

And:

> the sexual desires [in mental defectives] are exaggerated in proportion to the animal over the physic forces . . . the organs of reproduction are fully developed, in men they are even enlarged.[50]

Sterilisation was strongly recommended by the vast majority of physicians, psychologists and social workers, gaining widespread acceptance because proponents stated it was based on scientific principles. As with the earlier debates, it was again suggested that certain people carried 'bad seeds' and eugenicists used this position to advocate the *reproductive control* of these people. For eugenicists poor breeding resulted in 'mental retards', the 'mentally ill', epileptics, alcoholics and those with a tendency towards criminality. People deemed as 'good stock' on the other hand were encouraged to pass on their superior genes by having large families.[51]

In the United States of America far-reaching proposals were introduced to control 'defectives' and keep the race pure. One such proposal was the control of immigration into the country in order to preserve the nation's good stock. Another suggested the need to control marriage by passing laws that discriminated against certain socially undesirable groups. Many states passed laws that discriminated against these groups while other states went further and banned interracial marriages. This prohibition was enshrined in the *Miscegenation Laws,* the principles of which stated that mixing races produced inferior offspring, and it was not until the Civil Rights Movement of the 1960s that the laws were finally repealed. The same rationale applied to the institutionalisation of people deemed 'mental retards'. Many individuals in favour of institutionalisation said 'mental retards' had a 'right' to be institutionalised. Joseph Mastin, secretary of the Virginia Board of Charities and Corrections, highlighted this belief when in 1916 he wrote:

> The right of the defective, then, is not the right to live as he pleases, but the right to live the fullest life possible under proper guidance. But the right is just as sacred as our own and we must see that he has it; to deny it is a social crime as well as a violation of the commandment, "Thou shalt love thy neighbour as thyself." . . . Therefore, while mental defectives are clearly not entitled to the rights of normal persons, it is indisputable that society is under obligations to give them such training as may be suited to their needs and capacities. As a rule, mental defectives are descended from the poorer classes, and for generations their people have lived in homes having few conveniences. To expect them to be contented in a great city institution with its up-to-date furnishings and equipment . . . is unreasonable. When the State shall demand that those in charge of her degenerate and helpless people shall see that they live happy and useful lives and that procreation by them is rendered impossible: then we can look forward with confidence to the coming era when the feeble-minded will become extinct, mental disease will vanish and crime and pauperism will be reduced to a minimum. Then, and not until then, shall we get a clearer vision of the new heaven and the new earth wherein dwelleth *righteousness*.[52]

Eugenics and the Nazis' policy towards subnormals 1933–45

In Germany Hitler came to power in 1933, soon after which the Nazi Party began to put its vision of a biologically pure 'Aryan master race' into action. It was enshrined in law when on 14 July 1933 the Law for the Prevention of Progeny with Hereditary Disease was passed. The law forced the sterilisation of all persons who suffered from diseases considered hereditary, among whom were 'retards', those with 'congenital feeble-mindedness', as well as those suffering from 'mental illness', physical deformity, epilepsy, blindness, deafness and alcoholism. The general desire to eliminate illness and handicap from the population reflected, not only the political thinking of the day, but also the prevalent scientific and medical approaches. Germany remains the only country in history to carry out a mass sterilisation programme. The forced sterilisations began in January 1934 involving an estimated 300,000 to 400,000. Several thousand people died as a result of the operation itself, more women than men primarily because of the danger attached to the legation of ovarian tubes. Anyone considered feeble-minded provided the grounds for sterilisation and the vast majority of people were patients from mental hospitals and mental handicapped institutions. As a result of the 'Sterilisation Law' the Nazi regime set up 'hereditary health courts' which at their peak totalled 200 across Germany. The courts were made up of two physicians and a district judge; also local doctors were required to register with these courts any known cases of hereditary illness. Although appeal courts were established few decisions were ever reversed. In the rare event that an individual was given an exemption it was usually on the grounds that the person was a talented artist, for example, afflicted with mental illness. The Sterilisation Law was followed in 1935 by the Marriage Law which required for all marriages proof that any offspring would not be handicapped, disabled or suffer any other hereditary disease. One method used by the state to ensure this was a blood test prior to marriage.

The programme of forced sterilisation in Germany proved to be the forerunner for the systematic killing of 'subnormals', and in October 1939 Hitler initiated a decree that gave physicians the power to grant 'mercy deaths' to the 'retards'. The intention behind this programme of euthanasia was not to relieve the suffering of the chronically ill, but to exterminate the 'retards' and so cleanse the Aryan race of the 'genetically defective' and those who caused society a financial burden.[53] Propaganda helped to ensure the effectiveness of the campaign: mainstream cinema of the day stigmatised 'retards' by dwelling on the cost of caring for such individuals portrayed through special lighting effects as semi-human. The popular film *Das Erbe* ('Inheritance') is a notable example. In schools maths textbooks included questions such as 'The construction of a lunatic asylum costs 6 million marks; how many houses at 15,000 marks each could have been built for that amount?'[54]

The idea of killing 'subnormals' and 'retards' had first been presented as early as 1920 in a book co-written by Alfred Hoche, an eminent psychiatrist, and Karl Binding, a prominent scholar of criminal law. In their book *The Release of the Destruction of Life Devoid of Life*[55] they favoured the disposal of the 'unfit' suggesting the killing of 'useless lives' is justified in terms of economic savings. It was an idea that had originated from the economic deprivation experienced during and after the First World War. During that time many people in institutions had ranked low on the list for the rationing of food and medical supplies resulting in many starving to death or dying from disease. The First World War also had the long-term effect of undermining the value attached to individual human life, and the inter-war years saw hard times with a sharpening of economic policy especially where the 'undeserving' poor were concerned.

The Nazis began a regime of killing inmates in asylums and institutions but the party was fearful of public reaction, so, unlike the programme of sterilisation, these executions were carried out in secret. The code name given to these killings was *Operation T4*, a reference to Tiergartenstrasse 4 (Action T4) which was the address of the Berlin Chancellery Offices, the headquarters for the programme. T4 targeted adult patients in all government asylums, nursing homes and church-run sanatoria. The institutions were instructed to collect data via questionnaires about the state of health and capacity for work of all the patients. The completed forms were sent to expert assessors, made up usually of psychiatrists, who formed 'review commissions'. These experts marked each name with a plus sign in red pencil which meant 'death' or a minus sign in blue meaning 'allowed to live'. At first patients were killed by lethal injection, but by 1939 this had changed to mass killing by carbon monoxide gassing. The first gassings were carried out at Brandenburg Prison where gas chambers were disguised as showers complete with fake nozzles as a way of deceiving victims, and were the early prototypes for the later extermination camps. Meticulous records found after the war document the gassing of 70,273 individuals in six 'euthanasia' centres between January 1940 and August 1941. This total includes 5,000 Jews. Jewish 'subnormals' were killed regardless of their ability to work or their degree of disability, and records also showed the estimated savings made from these killings.[56]

Despite precautions by the Nazis it was not long before the secrecy surrounding Operation T4 broke down due to simple errors. For instance, in one case when the family asked about the circumstances surrounding the death, they were told that the person had died as a result of appendicitis; in fact the individual's appendix had been removed years before. Hairpins turned up in urns sent to the relatives of male victims, and thick smoke was clearly visible every day over Hadamar Crematorium where, in 1941, staff celebrated the cremation of the 10,000th 'retard' with beer and wine served in the crematorium. On 24 August 1941, and bowing to public pressure, Hitler ordered a halt to Operation T4. He ordered that the gas chambers from some euthanasia centres be dismantled and shipped to Poland. Later they were rebuilt and used for the 'final solution to the Jewish question'.

The killing of 'subnormals' did not, however, stop: the Nazi regime continued to send the message to doctors and psychiatrists that such people were *'useless eaters'* and *'life unworthy of life'*.[57] Doctors were encouraged to decide on their own who should live and who would die. The killing of 'mental defectives' became a normal part of hospital routine as infants, children and adults were put to death by starvation, poisoning and injection. Killings continued even after the Allied troops occupied Germany. In Kaufbeuren, for example, it was reported that killings in asylums continued for weeks after occupation. The same was true outside Germany in occupied territories like Poland, Russia and East Prussia where the death squads killed quite literally thousands of 'mental retards'. It is estimated that in all between 200,000 and 250,000 mentally and physically handicapped people were killed between 1939 and 1945 under the euthanasia and T4 programmes.

Only the Catholic Church within Germany voiced opposition to the sterilisation programmes on the grounds of Catholic doctrine. Clemens August, Count von Galen, Bishop of Munster, protested against the T4 killings in a sermon on 13 August 1941. Thousands of copies of his sermon were printed and circulated, but Hitler could not punish Galen because he ran the risk of openly and publicly clashing with the Catholic Church.

The new eugenics

At the beginning of this new millennium, there are an estimated 1.2 million people with learning disabilities in Britain. The range of learning disabilities varies from mild to profound and currently it is estimated that in the UK 200,000 adults and 50,000 children are classified as having severe or profound learning disabilities.[58] Many of these individuals have additional disabilities such as sight loss, hearing impairment, or restricted mobility, and one in three has some form of speech and communication difficulty. In more recent years the term 'dual diagnosis' has entered the language, becoming common among professionals who recognise that many individuals also have mental health problems. It is estimated that a quarter of a million adults and children in this country will need lifelong care and support, 25 per cent of whom suffer from profound multiple disabilities. Of the disabled children, 90 per cent live with their parents at home while 125,000 adults with profound disabilities also live with and are dependent on their families.[59] More recent statistical information published about the numbers and age ranges of people with a learning disability in Britain is presented in Figure 1.

Attitudes towards people with learning disabilities reveal remarkable variations adopted by the scientific, medical and social approaches. The literature highlights the different perspectives which can be seen clearly reflected through the use of language with terms such as 'incompatible approach', 'inconsistent categories' or 'ambiguous concepts'. Fryers (1997) believes that:

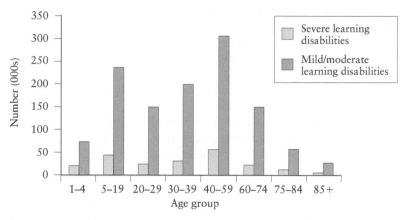

Source: Department of Health, *Valuing People: a New Strategy for Learning Disability for the 21st Century*. White Paper, Cm 5086 (London: HMSO, 2001)

Figure 1 People with learning disabilities, 1999

> Several equally important elements are difficult to reconcile in one taxonomy; genetic potential, aetiological diagnosis, brain damage and disorder, low measured intelligence, and social maladaptation. Each alone poses serious problems of classification, standardisation and measurement; together the difficulties are insuperable.[60]

Care professionals take all measures possible to avoid labelling people with learning disabilities; however, the scientific and medical communities have little problem categorising different groups under different labels. In fact quite the opposite is the case because they take the position that labelling is an essential part of treatment. Fryers suggests:

> . . . most cultures use social labels which are either stigmatising or promoted specifically because they are considered non-stigmatising . . . This should not affect professional[s] . . . although care professionals and researchers need to be aware of the differences between lay and professional language.[61]

There has been little agreement on terminology between scientific, health and social care professions because of the marked difference in approaches by each group, and they find it impossible to accommodate one set of terms of reference acceptable to all. The World Health Organisation (WHO) offered a definition it hoped would be acceptable to practitioners regardless of their field. In *International Classification of Impairments, Disabilities and Handicaps,* published in 1980, it presented the following structure.

> Impairment is a fault in an organ or body system; disability is a loss of function normal for any human being; handicap is social disadvantage

accruing from the impairment and disability. These can be applied to define mental retardation as a whole *(global categories)*,[62] or to define groups which have an important but not exclusive relationship with mental retardation (partial categories).[63]

Fryers examines 'Global categories', also referred to as 'Global learning disabilities', which are internationally recognised meanings that include: intellectual impairment, generalised learning disability and general dependency handicap. The first of these, intellectual impairment, is measured by intellectual testing through the intelligence quotient (IQ). Fryers observes that:

> ... many individuals with intellectual impairment are identified as learning disabled at school, but most are not regarded as mentally retarded adults [and that] mild mental handicap or retardation is always socially determined through IQ.[64]

It is interesting that as social services gradually began to take the lead responsibility from health the numbers of people identified as having 'mild mental handicap' became significantly reduced. The probable explanation was that social workers did not label people in the same way that medical and scientific professions have done in the past. Of underlying importance is that people are much more likely to be classified as having learning disabilities by social workers if they have communication problems, an additional physical disability, some form of challenging behaviour or a history of dual diagnosis. Classification can be described under a number of different headings, illustrations of which are summarised in Table 2.

During the last few years there has been a growing nervousness and unease with the emergence of studies into the genetical make-up of man and what has been referred to as the *new eugenics*. Dr Simonds was the first American physician who was active in establishing a *surrogate pregnancy*; when asked to justify his actions he replied: 'I performed the insemination because there are enough unwanted children and children of *poor genetic background* in the world.[65] Astonishing as Dr Simonds's remarks about reproduction may appear to us, with his unapologetic and clear use of eugenic language, it must come as no surprise to find his views are widely shared. For most of the last century, reproductive technologies have been about establishing the *superior* and reducing the *inferior*. One of the most prominent literary figures of the last century George Bernard Shaw, was excited by the prospect that artificial insemination offered the chance for multiplying the offspring of the gifted few. He wrote:

> When I, who have no children, and couldn't have been bothered with them, think of the ova I might have inseminated!!!! And all of the

Table 2 Factors affecting selection as mentally handicapped

Factor	Description
Legislation:	criminal, health, education, social welfare and employment law all relevant
Service structures and traditions:	in education, health, social welfare, etc.
Professional cultures:	concepts, perceptions, expectations, labelling, etc.
Patterns of employment and unemployment:	work and training opportunities
Social class and social attitudes:	cultural expectations, deprivation, discrimination
Family support:	structures and security of families
Historical service patterns:	older people inherited from earlier situations, e.g. in institutional care
Perceived low intelligence:	with or without additional factors, e.g. anti-social behaviour, mental illness, motor, sensory or communication disabilities, multiple disabilities
Certain medical diagnoses:	especially Down's Syndrome

Source: T. Fryers, 'Impairment, Disability and Handicap: Categories and Classifications', in *Seminars in the Psychiatry of Learning Disabilities*, ed. Oliver Russell (London: Gaskell and the Royal College of Psychiatrists, 1997), p. 28.

women who could not have tolerated me in the house for a day, but would have liked some of my qualities for their children!!![66]

Donor insemination has been used in Britain since the early 1930s, but unlike the German experience it has avoided provoking the same kind of anxiety. However, during the past decade the science has advanced dramatically and seen technological innovations develop resulting in phenomena such as the cloning of 'Dolly the sheep'. What is changing is that technical advances and remarkable leaps have been made towards a greater understanding of DNA. Scientists have successfully identified around 3,000 distinct conditions transmitted genetically.[67] Clinical tests for screening make it possible to detect conditions in the unborn foetuses: Down's Syndrome, for example can now be detected in older women before birth, giving them the option to abort. Other techniques have been developed that can identify genetical disorders in adults who may not realise they carry defects that can be passed to their children. Because of these new technical advances in science new problems and ethical dilemmas have arisen. There is a growing debate that is polarising opinion in the disability movement. Professionals in the fields of medicine and social services, academics and disability activists are joining together to discuss how people with learning disabilities may be affected by future advancements in genetical engineering. At the heart of the discourse lie the complex questions about reproductive choices, disability rights and the rights of the unborn. There is mounting concern over the new genetics and the eugenic overtones that can clearly be heard in the plans scientists have for genetic screening, and the future use of genetics.

Currently, doctors can assess during pregnancy whether a foetus is at high risk of developing a number of conditions. The journalist Kendra Inman, writing in the *Guardian* newspaper (April 2000), concluded:

> Increasing understanding of the human genome[68] and of the part genes play in a range of diseases means genetic testing for a wider range of disorders could be available in the near future.[69]

The fear is that routine use of genetic testing will increasingly result in women choosing to terminate a pregnancy rather than risk giving birth to a child with learning disabilities or any other disabilities. Critics argue that a rush for genetic testing could be a push to rid society of people with learning disabilities. Tom Shakespeare, a disability and genetics specialist at Newcastle University, observes:

> The disability movement is struggling to reconcile support for a woman's right to terminate a pregnancy, on the grounds that the baby may suffer impairment, with support for the rights of disabled people.[70]

Many within the disability movement are not against genetic screening but do have concerns about the implications. Abortion on the grounds that the foetus has an impairment is a significant step, and it is often the case that doctors do not have enough information or experience on issues of disability to discuss with the woman, in an informed manner, reasons for continuing the pregnancy. Bill Albert, chair of the Council of Disabled People's International Committee, agrees, saying: 'doctors are well-versed in the medical side of a disability but know very little about living with impairment.'[71] The issues are so emotive and difficult that people need to be guided through the 'moral maze' argues Tom Shakespeare, who calls for a report that will help men and women make decisions that are right for them.

During the time of the Conservative government in Britain, 1979–97, there began a renewed interest in human behaviour, particularly the responsibility of individuals for social problems, and the biological basis for behaviour. Attempts were made to blame the less well-off as being the source of society's ills with certain groups singled out. Lone parents and teenage pregnancies were regarded as among the chief causes of poverty, while juvenile delinquents were blamed for the rise in inner city crime and violent behaviour. The emphasis of the 1980s was on financial growth and economic prosperity, the survival of the fittest in a competitive market-place, with a shift in favour of rolling back the welfare state. The genuine concern to find solutions to some genetical diseases was over-shadowed by a far greater concern to reduce public spending and ultimately public responsibility. The period saw disabled people returned from institutions to a community indifferent to their needs, without adequate resources to ensure a decent quality and standard of living.

An important question for the future of genetical investigation, currently being debated, is what will happen to the data collected. Will they be used to develop new treatments for those affected by genetical disorders, or will such knowledge become a burden with the potential to limit autonomy and individual choice? These questions demonstrate the pivotal role of medical practice and its relationship to technical advances, individual choice, and the status of the disabled. Steps are being taken to redress the balance with the setting up of the Human Genetics Commission, a body that will advise the government about genetics. This body is working on drawing up a programme to investigate the ethical implications of storing genetic information. Opponents such as Agnes Fletcher, parliamentary officer for RADAR,[72] have called for an introduction of legislation that will address discrimination on the grounds of genetic make-up; she suggests that 'discussion can only bring us closer together. We need to reach a consensus in order to create a campaign agenda.'[73]

Today eugenicists hope that future genetical engineering will eventually mean problematic genes can be replaced in the embryo, thus creating the highest genetic standard in humans. The vision is a world without disability, disease or delinquency. The concern surrounding the *new eugenics* is that the definition of 'unfit' may become a new forum for intolerance and prejudice. Speaking in Mencap's magazine *Viewpoint* a woman with learning disabilities sums up her fears for the future:

> 'I believe that in the future they are going to try and wipe out people with a learning disability and people with certain disabilities. They don't want us to exist. They don't realise the things we can give to society, a knowledge that we have. As a young woman a specialist persuaded me to be sterilised, wrongly warning me that any baby would be bound to have severe disabilities. Nobody really told me it was my choice ... I regret it because now I can't have a child of my own, and yes, I would have liked one. I hope that when people start making laws based on this new science they will talk to us at the same time.'[74]

Steve Jones, Professor of Genetics at the University of London, is a leading expert in his field and a strong critic against any move towards the new eugenics. He concludes:

> 'the more I find out about people the more I realise that science cannot justify denying people the right to have children. Eugenicists were not only morally wrong, they were also bad science.'[75]

THE NATIONAL HEALTH SERVICE AND THE PROBLEM OF COSTS

These worries have emerged in post-war Britain alongside an increasingly firm commitment to policies that stress the rights of people with learning disabilities as citizens.

Returning to the position taken by the USA and Germany on eugenics, the same period saw British inter-war policy as being substantially at variance, and the association of eugenics with enforced mass sterilisation reduced British attachment to eugenics, as did the later Nazi extermination policy. As a consequence in the period of post-war reconstruction and reform, the focus of policy in Britain was to develop service responses from the base provided by the Mental Health Act 1927, the Mental Deficiency Act 1927 and the Wood Committee Report 1929. This was going to prove to be a difficult task not least of all because of the isolation and separation from family life. David Barron was sent to Whixley Institution at the age of 13 in 1939, and would spend the next 16 years of his life as a patient there. The extract 'Life in a mental institution' is taken from the book David has written about his experiences.

Life in a mental institution

'After taking one glance round the ward I knew there and then I did not like it. The place seemed more like a prison than a ward and in one sense of the word that is more or less what it was as I was about to find out. The attendant in charge took me through two rooms which were both locked. He had to unlock the doors then lock them again behind us. It was a case of wherever you went a bunch of keys were needed before you could gain access.

When I realised where he was taking me I went all of a tremble as the mere thought of Ward One was bad enough for me. He unlocked the door and took me into the punishment ward. As he was leaving I fired a last desperate question. "What have I done wrong, Sir?" "You should know. It was you that tore the page out of the book, son."

With that he left. For that great misdemeanour I was kept in Ward One for as near as I can recollect, five months. It broke my heart when the superintendent came on his daily rounds. Although I would look pityingly at him as he walked round the dining table I was just wasting my time. To make matters worse he went on his holidays for three weeks and I had the impression he had forgotten I was there.

During my stay there I was punished but not to the extent of some of the other patients. I was not made to go and scrub the yard with a brick . . . I think it was on account of my age that I was spared this humiliation but I may be wrong. You may be wondering why patients could be subjected to such a degrading task without anything being done to stop it, but what could the patients do?'[77]

Lewis Smith has similar memories of his time at Brockhall Hospital, where his mother left him as a young boy in 1942: 'Lewis' is quoted from his story.

Lewis[78]

"Were they nice?"

"No! Mr. Green was alright but Mr. Johnson weren't, he kept punching and hitting me and belting me around, he used to do it to me on Hazelwood, he was dreadful to me was Mr. Johnson, he was on the staff of Brockhall, he was dreadful to me was Mr. Johnson [repeated in original] That's going back some years . . . I went from Ivywood to Hazelwood, I think that must have been in 1944. You see, when I was in Hazelwood Mr. Johnson would be punching and hitting me, throwing boots and shoes and coat hangers, he used to throw cold water at me and make me sit in the cold bath . . . he was a bad 'un him, a bad beggar, you know I never liked him. I'm away from that now you know. Those days will never happen again. [I was there] from 1942 to 1988, forty-six years, yes that'll be right. I was on all sorts of different wards."

Lewis's story was transcribed by his friend Mary Edwards who added:

"It is important to Lewis that everybody knows what happened to him at Brockhall Hospital, that he was mentally, physically and sexually abused for his forty-six years internment. He is a gentleman with great dignity, humour and compassion that, if we take the time out of our relentless schedules to listen to, we can learn and grow from."

The National Health Service Act 1946

Further moves towards developing a policy of care in the community came with the creation of the *National Health Service* in 1946. One consequence of this change resulted in care for the 'mentally handicapped' being brought in line with the mainstream health care provision of the day. During the late 1940s and the early 1950s new developments in drug treatment were beginning to emerge which played a significant role in allowing people to remain in the community. The introduction of new types of medication and especially psychotropic drugs meant that some degree of control over an individual's anti-social behaviour could be exercised through the use of tranquillisers. Around 1948, asylums began changing their names and many became specialist 'mental handicap' hospitals. At the same time local authorities were taking on new responsibilities for a range of services under section 28 of the National Health Services Act 1946. However, local authorities only had two main *statutory* duties aimed at helping 'mentally handicapped' people which were:

(1) the initial care and removal to hospital of persons dealt with under the Lunacy & Mental Treatment Act;
(2) the ascertainment and (where necessary) removal to institutions of 'mental defectives' and the supervision of these in the community, under the Mental Deficiency Act.[79]

It was not surprising that with budget restrictions local authorities were less than enthusiastic about funding new services to a group not regarded as a priority.

THE NATIONAL COUNCIL FOR CIVIL LIBERTIES 1951

In 1951, the National Council for Civil Liberties published a pamphlet called *50,000 Outside the Law*.[80] This publication drew attention to the lack of legal safeguards for people in institutions and together with this, and related areas of concern, had a large impetus for the setting up of the Royal Commission (1954–7). Evidence was presented by the National Council that provided an outstanding historical statement concerning service provision to 'mentally handicapped' people, and included proposals for the future development of services along with new principles for the delivery of services. This was aided through the use of case studies that highlighted some of the greatest problems to do with hospital provision. For example, the statement decries the lack of training facilities available to patients in institutions, stating that any training provided was less about getting the person ready for an independent life, and more about sustaining the institution. The statement observed that:

the institution is so dependent on patient labour that even if the Medical Superintendent believed that a large number of *high-grade* patients were qualified for release, it would be impossible for release to be granted without bringing the institution to a standstill.[81]

The National Council cited incidents where the liberty of patients was brought into question and suggested that in a number of cases the freedom of the patient had been determined by the superintendent. A primary concern was abuse and the extreme forms of control exercised by the staff over the patients, and the statement held up as evidence cases where patients were too afraid to tell anyone about the abuse they suffered at the hands of staff, mainly because they were frightened that they would never be released.[82] In the summary the statement rejected the old eugenic arguments for the confinement of the 'mentally handicapped' and instead set out a number of new proposals:

(1) As far as possible, the services which exist for the normal citizens who need social help of any kind, should be used to provide for the mental deficients. Where special services become necessary, they should exist as departments of the appropriate general service. The provision of all such facilities to be made compulsory and not left to the discretion of the local and central authorities. Conditions within such a service should be at least as good as those for people in comparable services for other sections of the community.

(2) . . . a wide variety of both day and residential services must be made available and the closest liaison should exist between the specialist services and the school, the family doctor and the rehabilitation services of the Ministry of Labour.

(3) Financial assistance to be based on the principles of need and should not be in the hands of the administration of the service.[83]

The final paragraph proposed a framework based on citizenship, individual rights and duties and mutuality for society's response in a civilised age.

The idiot, the imbecile and feeble-minded are an integral part of the human race; their existence constitutes an unspoken demand on us. The extent to which we guard their right to the fullest and most useful life, the extent to which we guarantee to them the maximum freedom which they can enjoy and the extent to which we help their families to give them the love they need, is a measure of the extent to which we ourselves are civilized.[84]

THE ROYAL COMMISSION ON MENTAL ILLNESS & MENTAL DEFICIENCY 1954–7

The Royal Commission on Mental Illness & Mental Deficiency, established in 1954, published and presented its report in May 1957.[85] The Royal Commission aimed to:

> . . . enquire, as regards England & Wales, into the existing law and administrative machinery governing the certification, detention, care (other than hospital care or treatment under the National Health Service Acts 1946–52), absence on trial or licence, discharge and supervision of persons who are or alleged to be suffering from mental illness or mental defect, other than Broadmoor patients; to consider as regards England & Wales, the extent to which it is now, or should be made, statutorily possible for such persons to be treated as voluntary patients, without certification; and to make recommendations.[86]

The 1954–7 commission was charged with investigating the legal and administrative framework within which institutions operated in order to suggest changes that might be made. The commission asked a number of questions such as: *How appropriate was institutional care for patients?* and *What were the cost and funding implications, and the capacity in relation to efficiency within institutions?* When the commission published its findings, in the form of a report, these terms of reference had been extended to include a whole range of discourses on 'mental distress'. The commission questioned the wider issues about the way in which the needs of people had to be met through institutional care, and the investigation, and subsequent comments, formed the basis for recommendations made by the commission for changes to both the legal and administrative structures of services to the 'mentally handicapped'.[87]

The Royal Commission of 1954–7 called for the integration of the administrative structure of social welfare and health services, proposing partnership working, so that mental health services became integrated into the existing health and welfare departments of the local authorities. This move, the commission argued, would enable care to be provided on the scale already made available to older people and those with physical disabilities. It further recommended a number of key changes such as:

- mental hospitals should be administered and operated in a similar way to general hospitals, developing outpatient facilities and domiciliary care;
- mental hospitals should be integrated with local authorities to provide a continuum of care;
- the legal procedures for admission based on the Lunacy Act of 1890 were outdated, and [it proposed] the abolition of the legal process for admission of 'mentally distressed' individuals to hospital.[88]

The commission said that these changes were proposed for good reasons, one of which was the hope that such changes would rid society of the stigma surrounding 'mentally handicapped' people and that, where possible, treatment would become more accessible. The Royal Commission recognised the need from time to time for the compulsory admission of some individuals who were a danger to themselves or to others. Many patients in hospital could live in the general community with relatives or friends, but the report failed to clarify what it meant by outside the hospital and the 'community'.[89] It further failed to answer the question of how potential services would provide help to households who had a member or members deemed to be 'mentally defective'. The Ministry of Health welcomed the findings of the commission published in 1957, and praised it for the effectiveness that joint working practices, and an increase in the range of services, could offer. It was somewhat less enthusiastic when it came to a commitment for funding the new initiatives.

THE MENTAL HEALTH ACT 1959

Based on the Royal Commission the government responded with the 1959 Mental Health Act which proposed, among other things, a move for 'mental health services' away from the domain of the institution and towards community-based care. It extended services previously available to those with sensory impairments and the "general classes of the physically handicapped" under Section 29 of the *National Assistance Act* 1948. The Act brought recognition that care in the home had become official government policy, and this was the first piece of legislation to introduce a distinction between 'mental disorders'. It contained four distinct categories headed '*Definition & Classification of Mental Disorder*', which were:

(1) Mental Disorder
(2) Severe Subnormality
(3) Subnormality
(4) Psychopathic Disorder.[90]

The legislation set out to establish a framework of complex networks and support systems that aimed at enabling people to move out of long-stay hospitals and live safely in the community. The network of resources proposed included the establishment of day centres, residential units, initially in the form of large hostels, employment services, staffed housing and the appointment of mental welfare officers.

The 1959 Act states that there was no reason to continue to treat people in hospital if they could be released into the community with the help of drugs. The policy, however, also sought to return people to the community in order to reduce costs and save money, and the most effective way to achieve this was to run down overall hospital provision. The policy of running down and closing hospitals found support in some of the most unlikely, but for the government the most helpful, places. The policy was seen as listening to and responding to pressure from the anti-institution movement of the late 1950s and early 1960s to close institutions, for example. The policy was also supported through a number of academic studies such as that of Goffman's *Asylums* published in 1961.[91] Goffman said that institutions had a certain pattern and regime that ultimately de-personalised and de-humanised the individual. Goffman argued against the need for institutions suggesting they did not build around the needs of the person but actually made people worse because they created a state of dependency.

One voice against the policy of care in the community in the 1960s was that of Richard Titmuss. Titmuss said it was no good discharging people into the community unless adequate resources were put into community services, and he argued that very little thought had been put into the policy on community care. Titmuss believed that careful planning needed to go into what types of services were to be provided and he questioned: *Where responsibilities would lie? Who would be responsible for what?* Titmuss was to prove an accurate prophet regarding the inadequacies of community care with its lack of planning and resources. A number of commentators have argued that this period turned out to be disastrous for the 'mentally handicapped' who came out of long-stay institutions and were re-housed in the community. Services that had been promised under the policy of community care failed to materialise, leaving vulnerable people with little or no provision. By 1974, for example, 60,000 fewer residents were living in large mental hospitals than had been the case in 1954, but very few services in the community were operating to meet their needs.[92] A study by Dexter and Harbert, in 1983,[93] revealed that at the time only 10,000 of the families in Britain that had a 'mentally handicapped' member, had received a home help service since 1978. Previously there had been the option of hospital care, but this rapidly diminished and places in residential care were limited because of cost. Often the only service offered to the majority of families was basic day care.

EARLY INNOVATIONS IN COMMUNITY CARE AND THEIR IMPACT ON FAMILY LIFE

Successive governments paid little political interest to the transfer of 'mentally handicapped' children from hospitals to the community. However, they were forced to take notice due to a series of high-profile scandals in the hospitals, which drew attention to a lack of adequate facilities and poor resources. Until these scandals occurred in the late 1960s and throughout the 1970s, research studies undertaken had little impact in terms of changing policy. (See Stainton, 1992.[94]) Parental pressure groups were at the fore of campaigning, voicing their opposition to and demanding the closure of long-stay hospitals. Intense pressure also came from other groups such as the Spastics Society and the Campaign for the Mentally Handicapped (CMH). During the mid-1970s it was estimated by the CMH that some 8,000 children were still in hospitals and they said that 'mentally handicapped' children in hospital were among the most deprived in Britain.[95] Service provision and the development of social policy towards families with 'mentally handicapped' children had experienced a chequered and varied history.

THE POLITICAL & ECONOMIC PLANNING (PEP) REPORT 1966

During the early 1960s a study was called for that would examine the social outcomes of changes in psychiatric practice, and assess the progress of care in the community for 'mentally handicapped people' and their families. An investigation was called for that would explore the impact on family life that resulted from having a 'mentally handicapped' member of the family living at home. Professor Tizard and Dr J. Grad had previously undertaken a similar type of survey, between May 1955 and January 1957, for the Medical Research Council.[96] Their new study, to be carried out between October 1963 and May 1964, and based in London, used the same methodological approach as the 1954–7 study had as a basis for the project, the findings of which were published in 1966.[97] The research examined the attitudes of professionals working in social service departments and investigated 250 'severely subnormal' individuals, 150 of whom were living at home with their families, while the remaining 100 lived in institutions. The study aimed to examine services that people living at home received and compare the findings with institutional care. The study also explored reasons for admission to an institution and offered some explanations as to why and how community care was failing in these circumstances. Tizard and Grad looked at institutional care, contrasting it with family care, and concluded that families who cared for their 'child' at home were much more likely to be penalised through a number of measures including:

- a dramatic lowering in their general standard of living;
- strain on the family due to the pressure caused by looking after the individual;
- social isolation;
- anxiety about the future.[98]

Despite this, when the two groups were compared, it was discovered that individuals living at home were less likely to suffer problems connected with their health and social well-being than those who lived in institutions. A second important finding, the study revealed, was that despite attempts to develop care in the community, admission to hospitals had actually continued to rise.[99] The following illustration offers some explanation as to why.

> *Barbara*, a fifty-year-old defective, living with an eighty-year-old mother in two rooms. Dependent on the practical and financial assistance of a cousin in her sixties living nearby. They were in serious difficulties when the cousin broke her leg and could not help support the household. Barbara is a sensible person and helps a good deal with the chores. Her mother is very distressed at the imminent possibility of her being forced to ask for Barbara's admission to hospital merely because of her financial need.[100]

Alongside the summary of the findings, a number of recommendations were made which it was hoped would help parents to maintain their family member at home. One recommendation, for example, strongly advocated that local authorities needed to do more to help families by making small improvements to services ranging from extra grants for clothing, to a laundry service for the incontinent as well as home domestic and nursing help. These services it argued were easy to provide and were cheap. Other proposals included the need for more adult training places, and another serious problem the report identified was the way in which services to people with a 'mental handicap' and their families were prioritised suggesting:

> . . . there is ample evidence in this study of the willingness of parents to look after their handicapped 'child' even against the odds of low income, overcrowded homes and their own poor health. To support their efforts and avoid unnecessary hospital admission is to the advantage of the community as well as of the families concerned.[101]

Local authority involvement

The PEP Report analysed parental attitudes towards local authority services. The results highlighted the fact that parents mostly wanted services that helped them in practical ways, such as holiday schemes and places at training centres, but they had little or no interest in professionals such as mental health welfare officers. In contrast when these officers were interviewed by the researchers they saw themselves, and their routine visits, as being supportive and important to the families. Interestingly, during the course of the research it was discovered that even though the officers visited families at home, they demonstrated a remarkable lack of knowledge when asked, about the actual problems each family faced.

Local authorities provided three main services administered by their health departments during this period.

(1) Short-term care

Short-term care, first authorised in 1952 by the Ministry of Health, allowed temporary admission, for a period of up to eight weeks, to an institution. At the time of the publication of the PEP Report in 1966, the provision had been extended to include a variety of care such as the use of private foster homes and voluntary organisations. The report revealed marked differences in the use of short-term care depending on the area of London in which the family lived. Some authorities had a policy whereby almost all the individuals were offered the opportunity of an annual holiday, while in other areas of London only a few people were sent on regular holidays.

(2) Special care units designed to meet training and educational needs

Individuals attending training and educational units generally did so because they had been assessed as unsuitable for education in mainstream schools. Many parents were resentful of this, and demonstrated considerable bitterness believing that their child had been unfairly and wrongly assessed. Many argued that their child had not been given a reasonable chance to show his or her educational potential or true ability. However, no evidence was found by the PEP Report to support the parents' beliefs. Among other criticisms parents had were problems with transport, especially about the time spent waiting. Some parents were angry that they had to wait for up to half an hour in freezing weather or rain with their 'delicate child' for transport to take them to and from training centres.[102]

(3) The involvement of welfare officers

The third service provided by local authorities were the welfare officers. Undoubtedly by the end of the 1950s and in the early 1960s professional attitudes were beginning to change towards those called 'mentally handicapped'. However, even at this point in time traces of the language of eugenics could still be found in some reports. At the end of a year working with one family, a welfare officer, for example, summarised her case notes by stating 'care and control adequate'.

The overall picture that emerged from the PEP Report pointed to a

> . . . lack of flexibility [that had resulted] from adherence to administrative procedures. The focus is not the subnormal person himself, and his family surroundings, although essential to his welfare, are too often not taken into account. The narrowness of this approach is serious because

social workers could provide the channel by which the need for improvements in practical services was made known . . . Unfortunately, social work with the mentally handicapped has been for many years regarded as low in status compared with some other branches of the profession such as child care and probation . . . partly because *investment in the subnormal, unlike the deprived child, has been regarded as wasted.*[103]

The PEP Report explored what happened in institutions and then compared how this related to the alternative community care. It suggested that the potential for serious neglect was very much in evidence, and said it was as important to improve existing services, as it was to develop services to help support those individuals living at home with their families. The report interestingly saw the question of *choice* as being that of the parent not the individual. Most parents saw institutional care as a last resort, and one mental welfare officer during his interview with the researcher said some parents would often conceal serious problems, because of a fear that their child would be admitted to an institution. Most families wanted to take care of their children themselves for as long as possible.

   The PEP Report concluded on a positive note suggesting that there had been a growing awareness of the rights of 'the mentally handicapped' since the findings of the original Tizard and Grad study in 1954–7. This, it argued, was reflected in the growth of services such as increased training places, more trained workers, and an increase in both holiday provision and residential care. The findings were published against a background of highly publicised scandals highlighting the serious neglect of care in institutions, and this was also the context within which Seebohm published his report two years later in 1968.

THE SEEBOHM REPORT 1968

The Seebohm Report sought a more effective administrative structure for the development of community-based services. It recommended a unification of existing local authority services into one single department that would provide a community-based family-orientated service available to all.[104] The report suggested a framework within which community care would be provided and, as a result of these suggestions, by the mid-1970s the administrative structures of the national mental health services had undergone a considerable transformation. The Seebohm Report was the first major report that directly addressed the issue of care *by* the community as opposed to care *in* the community. Seebohm sought to give a definition to 'community'.

   The term 'community' is usually understood to cover both the physical location and the common activity of a group of people. The definition of a community, however, or even of a neighbourhood, is increasingly difficult as society becomes more mobile and people belong to communities of common interest, influenced by their work, education or social activities as well as where they live. Thus, although traditionally the idea of a community has rested upon geographical locality, and this remains an important aspect of many communities today different members of a family may belong to different communities of interest as well as the same local neighbourhood. The notion of community implies the existence of a network of reciprocal social relationships, which among other things ensure mutual aid and give those who experience it a sense of well-being.[105]

Seebohm's vision of care by the community is one of an interweaving of social services provision with that of the informal sector complemented by voluntary sector care. He proposed that social service departments should take the lead in developing care in the community. Everyone at some stage is a consumer of these services and as such, his report argues, the consumer is important in contributing to service planning. Both the attraction and importance of these ideas for the future development of services to 'the mentally handicapped' had been reinforced by the nature of the scandals. However, any further development of embryonic specialist skills among workers developing and delivering care to 'mentally handicapped' people was brought to an end by the replacement of specialist welfare officers with generic social workers.

PAULINE MORRIS'S *PUT AWAY* (1969)[106]

The Seebohm Report's championing of the community as opposed to institutional provision received substantial reinforcement within a year of its publication. Pauline Morris published *Put Away*, her findings of a five-year study conducted into conditions within mental handicap hospitals in 1969. The study was based on research undertaken in a cross-national sample of 35 hospitals. Morris found many problems including a lack of contact between patients and their relatives, and related factors such as the isolation of the hospitals, both in physical terms (location) and in the attitude of the professionals (doctors, nurses, and administration staff). She also discovered a serious need for better staff training, and concluded that the manner in which staff treated patients was at best unkind and she described the overall conditions as *Dickensian and grotesque*.[107] Morris noted that staff often became obsessed with trivial daily routines like counting sheets and that such tasks became the 'core tasks' to the exclusion and neglect of patients.

A significant factor, the study highlighted, was the length of time patients had been living in the hospitals. Statistics revealed that in a sample of some 3,000 patients 75 per cent had been in hospital for *at least* five years.[108]

Morris found patients with profound disabilities had staff assigned to them who were less skilled, less valued and less well paid; thus workers with fewer skills were working with patients who had the greatest needs. She discovered, in much the same way Goffman had previously, that there were established *patterns of care* within hospitals that were both rigid and inflexible and she noted that these institutions were places that did not welcome advice from *outside* professionals, instead this was felt to be not only unhelpful but also irrelevant and intrusive. Morris identified three modes of working practice within 'mental handicap' hospitals at the time that attempted to justify relationships and authority between staff and patients. These were:

(1) *a colonial-like mentality* – this sought a rigid separation between staff and patients;
(2) *prefect and fag* – here certain patients were picked out who would perform tasks for staff such as chores or run errands;
(3) *parent/child model* – which was the practice amongst most staff.[109]

In her summary Morris described the buildings in which patients lived as decrepit and rundown, the majority having been built before 1900. The patients slept in dormitories accommodating 60 or more people, barrack-like in style, with little furniture beyond the patient's own bed, and often there were only a few inches between beds. Many hospitals lacked any sense of a homely atmosphere; for example, day rooms were large and impersonal, lavatories and baths totally lacked privacy. There were no objectives regarding specialist treatments beyond that of confinement and alleviating families of the responsibility, and hospitals lacked specialist trained staff, and nursing duties were often confined to people with the most demanding physical needs. One nurse to 16 patients was normal for an average day, and there was little evidence that professionals exchanged or even discussed ideas amongst themselves about the running of the hospitals.

Morris's study was important because it was the first in-depth research to reveal what life was like for 90 per cent of people with 'a mental handicap' living in long-stay mental handicap hospitals in 1969.[110] The study attacked basic failings within the hospital system and underlined the regimes that existed. When published, *Put Away* drew public attention, though interest was short-lived and no immediate changes were made to hospital practices.

There was one political voice who actively advocated for change: this was the Labour Minister Richard Crossman who supported improving the hospital system. Crossman injected more cash into the system and succeeded in setting up a Hospital Advisory Service; however, this was towards the end of the Labour term of office and in 1970 the Conservatives took power. Critics who compare the way patients were dealt with at the time *Put Away* was published and more recent practices towards service users, suggest that although new services have developed and new working relationships, these relationships are not necessarily any better than those of the past. In the climate of community care, relationships are often based on the unreal idea of *staff as friends* of users and *equal colleagues*. These new relationships seek to be more optimistic and equitable, but they also seek to gloss over the professional working boundaries and power relationships that most professionals argue must exist.

Townsend on *Put Away*

Townsend in his foreword to *Put Away* offers a theoretical explanation for Morris's findings, suggesting that society has a desire to set clear boundaries between the *normal* and the *subnormal*. Townsend felt that the study raised a crucial question to the development of the discourse which was: *Do we need to revise our conceptions of mental handicap and transform our method of treating it?*

On the basis of the findings he argued that the case for social segregation had been eliminated and questioned whether hospitals were in fact the right places for treatment, offering instead community care as a viable alternative. He said 'mentally handicapped people' as a socially structured group, in terms of personal incapacity, were defined as a group incapable of managing their own personal functions, such as household tasks or personal care, and these were to a large extent determined by the hospital culture.

THE HOWE REPORT 1969

The movement towards care in the community was eventually fuelled by concerns over the basic standards of care in many mental handicap hospitals. These concerns were confirmed when in 1969, following allegations by a nurse to a *News of the World* reporter, the government was forced to take action and investigate the claims. The result was the 1969 Howe Report on Ely Hospital, Cardiff.[111] It was a damning publication that highlighted serious staff mismanagement, misconduct and cruelty towards patients, alongside poor physical conditions and a lack of equipment. This was the first in a series of reports to be published critical of institutional care.

THE WATKINS COMMITTEE REPORT 1970

The Howe Report was closely followed a year later by that of the Watkins Committee, which published its findings on the treatment of 'mentally handicapped' patients at the Farleigh Hospital.[112] This report resulted in three male nurses being charged and subsequently convicted on grounds relating to the cruel treatment of patients. The report went on to reveal a catalogue of appalling administration, with grossly inadequate levels of staffing and resources especially around the needs of individuals with challenging behaviour and profound disabilities. The incoming Conservative government's response to the Watkins Committee Report was the publication in 1971 of a White Paper specifically dealing with services for 'mentally handicapped people'.

THE WHITE PAPER *BETTER SERVICES FOR THE MENTALLY HANDICAPPED* (1971)

The publication of the White Paper *Better Services for the Mentally Handicapped* (1971)[113] aimed to define and re-structure services to people with a 'mental handicap'. The White Paper suggested this could be achieved to some degree through the provision of day centres, a personal assessment of needs, training and other forms of therapy. It differed significantly in its approach to the development of services from previous work such as that of Seebohm, for example, because it advocated the need for an 'interweaving of statutory and informal care'.[114] The White Paper called for changes to services for 'mentally handicapped' people with more importance being placed on the role of the family. It stated that each handicapped person should be aided to live with his or her family as long as it did not impose an undue burden on the family. It recognised the importance of help from family and friends, neighbours and the voluntary services, and in a general sense this was a turning-point in that the literature from here begins to describe the family in terms of the *caring family* and the *main source* of care:

> Most parents are devoted to their handicapped children and wish to care for them and to help them to develop their full potential. About 80 per cent of severely handicapped adults – and a higher proportion of the most mildly handicapped – live at home. Their families need advice and many forms of help, most of which at present are rarely available.[115]

The White Paper advocated halving the number of hospital places and instead using residential places provided by local authorities. Critics were quick to point out the failure of the White Paper to identify the funding necessary for the development of these services, saying this had a seriously adverse effect on policy implementation. The government sought to answer its critics by suggesting joint funding between health and social services and in 1974, the NHS Reorganisation Act brought about procedures that would effectively enable joint planning to take place. The proposal was for the introduction of joint consultative committees that would be member-based and would have the responsibility of carrying forward policies of de-institutionalisation. An immediate problem, however, was recognised and again it was one of funding, but in 1976 the government introduced joint financing with the principal aim to act as a

. . . mechanism by which social service departments could obtain health authority money for a time limited period to fund community care initiatives, which would either make a contribution to the hospital run-down programme or provide support for people to remain in the community rather than to seek hospital entry.[116]

THE PAYNE REPORT 1972

In 1972 yet another report, the Payne Report of Inquiry, followed and once again it exposed neglect and the abuse of patients, this time at the Whittingham Hospital. The revelations about the treatment of patients by staff followed the same patterns as the previous inquiries with the Howe Report (1969) and the Watkins Committee Report (1970). Collectively, these reports had the effect of increasing public awareness while at the same time bringing substantial pressure for change to bear on politicians and policy makers. The need for change was now at the forefront of government policy and swift action was needed. Disability campaigners called on the government to produce policies more in line with the principles of ordinary life: they wanted equality by achieving the same rights for people with learning disabilities as the rest of society.

THE REPORT OF THE COMMITTEE OF ENQUIRY INTO MENTAL HANDICAP NURSING AND CARE: THE JAY REPORT 1979

One of the earliest indications that the principles of normalisation were beginning to influence social policy discourse, even at central government level, came with the publication of the *Report of the Committee of Enquiry into Mental Handicap Nursing and Care* (the Jay Report 1979). This report, amongst other things, called for a review of nurse training and proposed a new model of training in line with the philosophy of ordinary life. The report was very much influenced by the concept of normalisation and social integration. It was unusual as a report in that it began, not with a review of services, but with a philosophical debate on 'the rights of mentally handicapped people', and from this position developed the idea of an appropriate model of care. The main focus of the report emphasised the individual's right to a normal life stating that: 'mentally handicapped people have a right to enjoy *normal patterns of life* in the community.'[117]

It argued that the framework for services should be one that both respects the person using the services, and also meets that person's need. The Jay Report was critical of large institutional forms of care in the community, such as large hostels, on the grounds that housing people in purpose-built units on the outskirts of towns and cities did not promote participation in the community. It argued that 'mentally handicapped people' had the right to live in ordinary homes in ordinary streets, and like the 1971 White Paper emphasised that community care meant providing local services and accommodation in local settings. But the pursuit of such social integration was not without problems. Integration remained dependent on government funding for new and existing services to support individuals in the community. Yet government money often found more immediate priorities elsewhere. In practice the new Conservative administration of 1979 found its expenditure plans almost de-railed and the objective of keeping people in their own homes where possible thwarted by its attempt to stimulate the private market in residential care.

SOCIAL SECURITY FUNDING AND THE 'PERVERSE INCENTIVE'

During the 1980s a rapid growth took place in private residential homes and nursing homes. The DHSS changed the supplementary benefit regulations in 1983, to make it easier for residents of these homes to claim their fees from the social security system to encourage private market provision. Public subsidy was not based on an assessment of care needs, but rather on an assessment of financial entitlement only.[118]

The Conservative government grew concerned about the cost as the rapidly increasing bill threatened to undermine its policy of economic restraint through cuts in public expenditure. In 1979, for example, the amount spent stood at £10 million, in 1986 it was £459 million, and by 1991 it was an unbelievable £1,872 million p.a.[119] At the same time worries increased regarding the standards operating within residential care, and the demoralised state of those working in it, especially in the statutory sector. At a time when, for reasons of economy and good practice, the government wished to expand community-based domiciliary and daycare services, the system was encouraging both local and health authorities to place service users in residential homes.

THE INDEPENDENT REVIEW OF RESIDENTIAL CARE 1985

In 1985, the Secretary of State for Health and Social Services, Norman Fowler, established the *Independent Review of Residential Care* appointing Gillian Wagner as chair. The aim was to:

> ... review the role of residential care and the range of services in statutory, voluntary and private residential establishments within the personal social services in England and Wales.[120]

Wagner was a response to the need for effective regulation in the aftermath of 1983, and reflected a continuing concern over scandals. Interestingly, the main themes that emerged from the report are questions about *choice* and *rights*. Wagner writes:

> To give power of choice to the consumer is important because it changes the fundamental relationship between the client and the professional, and on a wider scale, between the dependent person and society.[121]

She continues:

> We have to recognize that there are people who, in differing degrees and for different reasons, are incapable of deciding for themselves; they include babies, [and] people with severe mental handicaps.[122]

Wagner explores the importance of family involvement in the decision-making process about services. However, because advocacy was only in its infancy, she has little to say about them, only mentioning advocates in the section dealing with the complaints process, a context in which they are considered to have value as arbitrators by virtue of their independence and impartiality, rather than as supporters of the interests of the service users, because of their impartiality and independence.[123] Wagner recommended having a nominated social worker for the client, whether a field social worker or a residential social worker is of little importance. What was important was for the person to be trained and act as an agent providing imaginative packages of care. The assessments must be needs-led and not resources-led. Wagner continues this theme by suggesting the adoption of the Kent community care model where social workers had budgetary control over the client's care package, which at the time was a contentious area of concern for the disability lobby.[124] Among other interesting proposals presented in her report is the early notion of direct payments: Wagner suggests that people with specific needs should be given a community care allowance with which to purchase services, arguing that the advantages of such a scheme are likely to include:

- making flexible community care provision;
- adopting such an approach would encourage individual choice;
- an outcome more satisfactory to the client as consumer.[125]

Wagner's Report is an example of a rights-based approach advocating the rights of people including those with a mental handicap. She is in favour of individual funding for the users and support for decision-making in personal planning. Mostly after the Wagner Committee began work, the government's policy was assailed from two important sources, the Social Services Committee of the House of Commons and the Audit Commission, which set in motion a train of events and led to the administrative restructuring of local authority social services provision.

THE HOUSE OF COMMONS SELECT COMMITTEE REPORT: SOCIAL SERVICES COMMITTEE 1985[126]

In 1985 the House of Commons Select Committee[127] began to examine service provision to adults with learning difficulties, drawing attention to a number of problems with community care policy:

(1) The policies did not highlight that the majority of people with special needs were already being cared for by their families at home.
(2) There was no agreed consensus on what constitutes 'good' community care.
(3) The report described a 'cart before the horse' syndrome in that hospital provision was being run down quicker than alternative community-based services were being put in place.
(4) Services had been under-financed and under-staffed. It was seen that joint financing meant little more, in practice, than the transfer of responsibility from the health to the local authority.
(5) *The consumer should have a voice in the creation and development of services.* There needed to be tighter arrangements in place for joint funding with a 'central bridging fund' for the transmission of moneys from one authority to the next.[128]

The government's reply to the critics was not what was either expected or welcomed. The statement was brief, rejecting the committee's recommendations for more resources to be put into basic services.

THE AUDIT COMMISSION REPORT: *MAKING A REALITY OF COMMUNITY CARE* 1986

Equally critical of the system in the mid to late 1980s was the Audit Commission Report *Making a Reality of Community Care* (1986a).[129] The report said that progress around moving people out of long-stay hospitals had been slow, and often people were simply moved from one form of institution to another, for example, out of hospital and into an old people's home, as opposed to a community-based service. The report identified what it suggested were the main problem areas. The first was a lack of co-ordination of services; this entailed confusion around the delivery of services and a fragmentation of responsibility. Secondly, it argued in favour of a bridging fund (which had already been established for learning difficulties under the All Wales Strategy 1983). Thirdly, social security policy came in for criticism because the system encouraged both the health and local authorities to place people in residential care and nursing homes rather than ordinary housing in the community – the 'perverse incentive'. Finally, it highlighted a serious lack of adequately trained staff. The Audit Commission called on central government for a review that would come to clear decisions about the future of community care. The government responded with the Griffiths Inquiry set up largely to investigate the problems created by policies, especially the perverse incentive.

Amongst the Griffiths Inquiry's strategic vision for community care was the appointment of a minister especially for community care, and national standards set by central government. Implementation of policy would remain the responsibility of local authorities, and each local authority would present a set of community care plans for approval by central government; and thus the role of central government would be limited to that of a monitoring function. As expected, Griffiths recommended that finance would come directly from central government to aid the development of community care.[130] Griffiths's main message was essentially that responsibility for community care must be placed with local authorities. This was contentious to a Conservative government whose whole approach towards local government was one of hostility with a clear agenda to reduce it. Griffiths said his recommendations would allow the consumer a wider choice because it would create flexibility and innovation, and would stimulate competition within service provision. To ensure this was so he further argued that social service providers should see themselves, not as monopolistic providers, but rather as arrangers and purchasers of care services to be provided by the voluntary and private sectors.[131] He agreed with Wagner's proposal for a care management system that would be responsible for assessing individual need, while also taking into account the views of family, friends and informal carers. The Griffiths approach and the advocacy of care management by Wagner had been pioneered by the Kent community care project under Bleddyn Davies.

Care packages would reflect need, but it would be up to the authority to 'determine the priority of the case, given the total resources available and the competing needs of others'.[132] One serious problem with Griffiths's proposals was the fact that total control is in the hands of the care manager (social workers) creating a potential conflict of interests. Griffiths suggested a single point of entry for both carers and consumers of services. Wagner was also clear about the possibility of a conflict of interest when she proposed having the agent attached to the providing authority with responsibility for funding care packages. Griffiths argued that homes in the private, voluntary and public sectors should receive funding once a full assessment had been made on the individual, including financial *means* and *care* needs. These assessments were to be carried out separately but managed by social services, and each assessment would begin by looking at the accommodation that would most appropriately meet the needs of the individual. After the initial stage a financial assessment was to be carried out by social security. The residential allowance would be set, taking into account the average total income, including income support and housing benefit for an individual living in other than a residential home, with the balance made up by social security.

RESPONSES TO THE GRIFFITHS REPORT 1989

The government's response to the Griffiths recommendations was set out in the 1989 White Paper on Community Care, outlining a new funding system for those seeking support for residential or nursing home placements. The local authority would take on the responsibility for funding placements in homes, made possible by the transfer of moneys from the social security budget to local authorities. Local authorities could use the money to fund domiciliary care, or residential services as they saw fit.

The White Paper *Caring for People: Community Care in the Next Decade and Beyond* (1989)

In November 1989, the White Paper *Caring for People: Community Care in the Next Decade and Beyond* was published based on the Griffiths recommendations. The White Paper was intended as a review of policy and examined the future direction policy should take. The government was forced to acknowledge the failings of the previous community care policy and the problems caused by the 'perverse incentive'. It also had to acknowledge the need for services to expand, particularly in areas such as supporting the needs of the carers, and targeting the needs of minority ethnic groups. The White Paper accepted earlier criticisms about the way in which hospitals had been run down and closed without prior and adequate provision being put in place before patients were discharged. However, the overall tone of *Caring for People* was one of optimism as it proposed new measures to combat criticisms. Among these proposals was the transferring of funds from the social security budget that would allow for an increase in smaller residential-type settings, and an expansion of supported living schemes as well as more domiciliary care. Greater importance was also given to the not-for-profit sector and informal care recognising a need for greater co-ordination of services. Improving efficiency is a key theme running throughout the White Paper, and seeks to achieve greater efficiency by providing specialist services. However, ambiguity is evident when it comes to finance; for example, in paragraph 7.5 we are told:

> The Government recognises that progress has not been uniformly satisfactory and there are legitimate concerns that in some places hospital

beds have been closed before better, alternative facilities were fully in place. Some reports also suggest that, at times, patients have been discharged without adequate planning to meet their needs in the community . . . Ministers will not approve the closure of any hospitals unless it can be demonstrated that adequate alternatives have been developed.

This approach appears at odds with a later statement (para. 7.10):

Finance from the sale of mental illness and mental handicap hospitals can provide valuable capital for replacement facilities.[133]

The recommendations argued that the proposals provided sound financial structures on which good-quality community services could be delivered through clear systems of management that separated social care from medical treatment.[134] The government argued this was the strength of the White Paper because it separated out *treatment* from *care*. Care became the social and community responsibility, while treatment lay in the hands of the NHS. The White Paper followed a number of proposals put forward by Griffiths. Social services departments would continue in their lead role, arranging and purchasing care, but without being monopolistic or dominant providers of care. Choice for users was regarded as a priority, to be encouraged by the use of the voluntary and private sectors in so far as their services represented a '*cost effective care choice*'.[135] It continued by detailing the main responsibilities local authorities would have as lead agents including:

- The assessment of individual need which would look at the social, educational and housing need of the individual, to be carried out in association with other agencies; medical, nursing and so on, before reaching a decision about appropriate services for the person.
- The appointment of a care manager who would design a care package tailored to individual need taking into account the needs of the carer.
- [They would] become enabling authorities through a combination of purchasing and providing services including the contracting out of services, with a clear split between the two roles.[136]

The government said that through the care management system, social services would be in a better position to deliver needs-led rather than service-led services. The requirement on social service departments was to produce community care plans, in line with those of the health authority, which would be subjected to a yearly inspection by the Social Services Inspectorate. The plans needed to demonstrate the ways in which social service departments had maximised their use of voluntary sector services, and the White Paper included three other major changes to the system:

- the introduction of a complaints procedure;

- a new inspection department to be set up which would be separate from the main body of the social services department, but accountable to the director of social services.
- financial support for individuals in private residential and nursing homes, to become the responsibility of social service departments. Money could also be used to finance domiciliary care and thus reduce the numbers going into residential homes.

In the spirit of the Griffiths Report, local authorities were encouraged to meet the needs of the client through flexible packages of care. The plans would explain how services could successfully be expanded and developed. From here on, the jargon of 'the market-place' – that of choice and consumer participation for social care provision – was becoming well and truly established through a *mixed economy of care*. The buzzword became 'diversification' with a diversity of services to suit all, but critics argued this was nothing more than a weak Tory ploy for the *marketisation* of public services. Public services would be contracted out with little guarantee that there would be adequate public resources or quality provision. Notably absent from the White Paper were the Griffiths recommendations for ring-fenced funding and a minister for community care.

SUMMARY

This chapter recounts the movement of social policy through Acts of Parliament and government legislation, examining how they have shaped services to people with learning disabilities. Moving through history an understanding is given as to how and why present-day community care has evolved in the way it has. The historical controls on the lives of people with learning disabilities, throughout the ages, such as those of Church and State, have been explored. The ability of social policy to change lives is demonstrated, while at the same time the contradictions and tensions are highlighted through the central themes the book seeks to examine including those of: normalisation, empowerment, and choice contrasted against the reality of government funding to social services departments.

The Political and Economic Planning Report (PEP) 1966 links old ideas of paternalism and control to the new beginnings of community care, and evaluates a significant change in social policy and working practice. Pauline Morris in *Put Away* draws her reader to ask the same moral question as Townsend when he asks: *'Do we need to revise our conceptions of mental handicap and transform our method of treating?'*

Other themes of equal importance which emerge through this chapter, and which will be examined in greater detail later on in the book are those of:

- professional relationships;
- relationships between the statutory agency and voluntary sector; and relationships between the statutory agency and the family;
- partnership working;
- problems of defining and rationalising diversity.

This book is going to consider the empirical work, but also in a more general sense ethical and professional questions.

NOTES

3 Plato, *The Republic*, 2nd edn, trans. Desmond Lee (Harmondsworth: Penguin, 1974), pp. 240–1. 'Guardians' is the term Plato uses for his ruling elite.
4 Aristotle, *The Politics*, revised T. J. Saunders, trans. T. A. Sinclair (Harmondsworth: Penguin, 1981) p. 439.
5 Plato, *Republic*, p. 241.
6 W. T. Jones, *A History of Western Philosophy*, Vol. I, *The Classical Mind*, 2nd edn (New York: Harcourt Brace Jovanovich, 1970), pp. 238–9.
7 Aristotle, *De Anima*, trans. Hugh Lawson-Tancred (Harmonsworth: Penguin, 1986), pp. 197–8.
8 The terms by which people with learning disabilities are referred to such as 'idiot', 'fool', 'retard', 'mentally handicapped' and 'learning difficulties' are used within their historical context.
9 Timothy Stainton, *Autonomy & Social Policy: With Special Reference to Mental Handicap in Ontario and Britain* (Ashgate Publishing: Aldershot, 1994; Brookfield, VT: Avebury, C.), p. 150.
10 B. B. Warfield, "Introductory Essay on Augustine and the Pelagian Controversy", in *A Select Library of the Nicene and Post-Nicene Fathers of the Christian Church*, Vol. 5: *Saint Augustin: Anti-Pelagian Writings*, ed. Philip Schaff (Grand Rapids: Wm B. Eerdmans, 1956).
11 ibid., pp. 27–8.
12 Paracelsus (1493–1541), more properly, Theophrastus Phillippus Aureolus Bombastus von Hohenheim, was one of the most important Renaissance naturalists and a towering figure of importance in his age. He was associated with the shattering of medieval thought and the birth of the modern world. Scientific debates of the late 16th century were centred frequently on the innovations of Paracelsus. Internet: "Philippe Pinel" – encyclopaedia article from Britannica.com http://www.britannica.com/seo/p/philippe-pinel/
13 Paul F. Cranefield and Walter Federn, "The Begetting of Fools: An Annotated Translation of Paracelsus' DE GENARTIONE STULTORUM", *Bulletin of the History of Medicine* 41 (1967): 161–74.
14 ibid., pp. 70–2.
15 Cited in R. C. Scheerenberger, *A History of Mental Retardation* (Baltimore, MD: Paul H. Brookes, 1983), p. 36.
16 'Phippe Pinel', http://www.britannica.com/seo/p/philippe-pinel/
17 Michel Foucault, *Madness and Civilisation: A History of Insanity in the Age of Reason* (London: Tavistock, 1967), p. 242.
18 Charles Tylor (ed.), *Samuel Tuke (1784–1857): His Life, Work and Thoughts* (London: Headley, 1990).
19 Quakers have always held the belief that there is 'that of God' in every human being. The 'promptings of love and truth' are heard from the heart and Quakers

refer to this, not just as conscience, but as *'the Inner Light'*, or *'the Voice of God'*, or *'the Light of Christ Within'*. They share the same principle: that of respect for the Light within each person. For further references see the internet: 'Quaker Views – Introduction: Making Decisions' and 'A Glossary of Quaker Terms': http://www.quaker.org.uk/more/qviews/qviews1.html

20 Kathleen Jones, *Asylums & After: a Revised History of the Mental Health Services: from the Early 18th Century to the 1900s* (London: Athlone Press, 1993), p. 26.

21 See the internet: "The Final Struggle and the Victory of Science – Pinel and Tuke": http://www.santafe.edu

22 G. Sutherland, with Stephen Sharp, *Ability, Merit and Measurement: Mental Testing and English Education* (Oxford: Clarendon Press, 1984), p. 29.

23 Tylor, Samuel Tuke (1784–1857); p. 312.

24 ibid., p. 313.

25 The Idiots Act, Parliamentary Papers, Vol. II (1886).

26 Stainton, *Autonomy & Social Policy*, p. 178.

27 J. L. Down, 'Classification of Idiots, Clinical Lecture Reports, London Hospital' (1866), in Leo Kanner, *The History of the Care and the Study of the Mentally Retarded* (Springfield: Charles C. Thomas, 1964); cited in ibid., pp. 103–4. Scheerenberger, *A History of Mental Retardation*, p. 57.

28 P. Williams, 'The Nature and Foundations of the Concept of Normalisation', in E. Kracas (ed.) *Current Issues in Clinical Psychology 2* (New York: Penguin, 1985).

29 F. Galton, *Hereditary Genius: An Inquiry into Its Laws and Consequences* (London: Macmillan, 1892 [1869]).

30 F. Galton, *Inquiries into Human Faculty and Its Development* (London: Macmillan, 1883).

31 "Eugenics." http://www.encarta.msm.com/find/concise

32 N. Malin, D. Race and G. Jones, *Services for the Mentally Handicapped in Britain* (London: Croom Helm, 1980), p. 43.

33 E. Goffman, *Asylums: Essays on the Social Situation of Mental Patients and Other Inmates* (Harmondsworth: Penguin, 1968).

34 Foucault, *Madness and Civilisation*, p. 31.

35 Andrew Scull, *Museums of Madness: The Social Organisation of Insanity in Nineteenth-Century England* (London: Allen Lane, 1979).

36 Peter McIntyre, 'Is this the new genetic science eugenics in disguise?', *Viewpoint*, no. 59 (June/July 2001): 3.

37 D. Galdstone, 'The Changing Dynamics of Institutional Care: The Western Counties Idiot Asylum 1864–1914', in D. Wright and A. Digby (eds), *From Idiocy to Mental Deficiency: Historical Perspectives on People with Learning Disabilities* (London: Routledge, 1996), p. 138.

38 *Western Counties Asylums Annual Report* (Exeter: Northcott Devon Medical Foundation, 1902), p. 16.

39 M. Oswin, 'An Historical Perspective', in C. Robinson and K. Stalker (eds), *Growing up with Disability* (London: Jessica Kingsley, 1998).

40 Caroline MacKeith, 'A Young Woman's Diary from 1901', in *Telling Our Own Stories: Reflections on Family Life in a Disabling World*, Pippa Murray and Jill Penman (eds) (Sheffield: Parents With Attitude, 2000), pp. 7–13.

41 G. R. Searle, 'Eugenics and Class', in *Biology, Medicine and Society 1840–1940*, ed. Charles Webster (Cambridge University Press, 1981), p. 9.

42 *Royal Commission on the Care and Control of the Feeble-Minded, Minutes of Evidence*, Vols I–VII, *Report*, Vol. VIII. Parliamentary Papers, Vols XXXV–XXXIX (1908).

43 ibid., p. 1.

44 ibid., p. 7.
45 A. F. Tredgold, 'The Feebleminded – a Social Danger', *Eugenics Review* 1 (London: 1909): 97–104.
46 ibid., p. 105.
47 A. F. Tredgold, Assisted by R. F. Tredgold, *A Textbook on Mental Deficiency (Amentia)* (London: 1952).
48 Internet: "Handicapped" published by the United States Holocaust Memorial Museum. http://www.ushmm.org
49 G. Shuttleworth, *Mentally Deficient Children: Their Treatment and Training* (London: H. K. Lewis, 1985).
50 M. Barr and E. Maloney, *1921 Types of Mental Defectives* (London: P. Blakiston, 1904).
51 David Smith, *Pieces of Purgatory: Mental Retardation in and out of Institutions* (Belmonth, CA: Brooks/Cole, 1995), pp. 73–5.
52 ibid., pp. 77–8.
53 Internet: "Handicapped". http://www.ushmm.org.
54 ibid.
55 K. Binding and A. Hoche, *The Release of the Destruction of Life Devoid of Life* (Leipzig: F. Meiner, 1920).
56 Internet: "Handicapped". http://www.ushmm.org
57 James M. Glass, *Life Unworthy of Life: Racial Phobia and Mass Murder in Hitler's Germany* (New York: Basic Books, 1997).
58 Internet: "What is Learning Disability?" http://www.mencap.org.uk
59 Department of Health, Valuing People; A New Strategy for Learning Disability for the 21st Century, A White Paper, Cm 5086, HMSO 2001, p. 15.
60 T. Fryers, 'Impairment, Disability and Handicap: Categories and Classifications', in *Seminars in the Psychiatry of Learning Disabilities*, ed. Oliver Russell (London: Gaskell and the Royal College of Psychiatrists, 1997), p. 19.
61 ibid., p.16.
62 Italics added by author.
63 World Health Organisation, *International Classification of Impairments, Disabilities and Handicaps* (Geneva: Fryers, 1980).
64 ibid., p. 19.
65 N. Keane and D. Breo, *The Surrogate Mother* (New York: Everest House, 1981), p. 36.
66 D. Kelves, *In the Name of Eugenics* (Harmondsworth: Penguin, 1986), pp. 191–2.
67 A. Breeching and J. Walmsley (eds), *Making Connections: Reflecting on the Lives and Experiences of People with Learning Difficulties: A Reader* (Milton Keynes: Open University, 1989), p. 89.
68 Researchers on the Human Genome Project have completed a draft of mankind's genetic code, an achievement being hailed as one of the greatest scientific feats. The £2 billion project has involved scientists from the United States, Britain, Germany, France, Japan and China. The government's chief adviser said: 'The Genome Project is a scientific development on a par with Charles Darwin's *Origin of Species*, and is probably a landmark more significant than man landing on the moon.' Supporters of the project suggest the eventual outcome could mean that doctors will be in a position to tell patients what chances they have of contracting diseases such as Alzheimer's and cancer. Genetic diseases not screened out during pregnancy would be treated at a later stage by gene therapy. Critics fear this could mean producing genetically modified children, but supporters dismiss this by saying the research will lead to major advances in the treatment of illness. Scientists acknowledge the most

lucrative benefits for this type of scientific research lie in the discovery of a 'cure' for ageing. A leading member of the government's Human Genetics Commission said 'advances in genetics would create a race of "immortals"'. He continued: 'We are contemplating a world in which future children would have to compete indefinitely with previous generations for jobs, space and everything else.' Metro, "On the Threshold of 'Immortal Mankind'", 26 June 2000 (London).

69 K. Inman "Testing Times", *Guardian*, 5 April 2000.
70 ibid.
71 ibid.
72 RADAR is the Royal Association for Disability and Rehabilitation.
73 Inman, 'Testing Times'.
74 McIntyre, ' Is this . . . Eugenics in Disguise?', p. 3.
75 ibid.
76 David Barron, 'Life in a Mental Institution', in *Telling Our Own Stories: Reflections on Family Life in a Disabling World,* Pippa Murray and Jill Penman (eds) (Sheffield: Parents with Attitude, 2000), pp. 14–15.
77 ibid.
78 Lewis Smith, "Lewis", in *Telling Our Own Stories: Reflections on Family Life in a Disabling World*, Pippa Murray and Jill Penman (eds) (Sheffield: Parents with Attitude, 2000), pp. 17–19.
79 E Murphy, *After the Asylums: Community Care for People with Mental Illness* (London: Faber & Faber, 1991).
80 National Council for Civil Liberties, *50,000 Outside the Law* (London: NCCL, 1951).
81 Royal Commission on the Law Relating to Mental Illness & Mental Deficiency 1954–1957, *Minutes of Evidence* (London: HMSO, 1957), p. 824.
82 ibid., pp. 827–8. and p. 832.
83 ibid., p. 851.
84 ibid., p. 854.
85 ibid., para. 3.
86 Cited in S. Goodwin, *Community Care and the Future of Mental Health Service Provision: Studies of Care in the Community,* 1st edn (Aldershot: Avebury Gower, 1990).
87 Royal Commission on the Law Relating to Mental Illness & Mental Deficiency, 1954–1957, *Minutes of Evidence,* para 3.
88 S. Goodwin. *Community Care,* p. 36.
89 Royal Commission on the Law Relating to Mental Illness & Mental Deficiency 1954–1957, *Report and Minutes of Evidence,* p. 592.
90 Department of Health, *Mental Health Act (Part 1 Section 4)* (London: HMSO, 1959).
91 E. Goffman, *Asylums: Essays on the Social Situation of Mental Patients and Other Inmates* (Harmondsworth: Penguin, 1968).
92 E. Murphy, *After the Asylums,* p. 60.
93 M. Dexter and W. Harbert, *The Home Help Service* (London: Tavistock, 1983).
94 Timothy Stainton, 'A Terrible Danger to the Race', *Community Living* 5(3) (January 1992): 18–20.
95 Campaign for the Mentally Handicapped, *Whose Children?* (London: CMH [now Values into Action], 1975), p. 9.
96 J. Tizard and J. C. Grad, *The Mentally Handicapped and Their Families,* Maudsley Monograph no. 9 (1961).
97 J. Moncrieff, *Mental Subnormality in London: A Survey of Community Care,* political and economic planning report (London: 1966).
98 ibid., p. 51.

99 Registrar-General, *Statistical Review of England & Wales* (1960) *Supplement on Mental Health, Report of the Committee on Local Authority Personal Social Services* (the Seebohm Report), Home Office Department of Education & Science, Ministry of Health (1968). Cmnd 3703. (London: HMSO, 1960).

100 J. Moncrieff, *Mental Subnormality*, p. 33.

101 ibid., p. 52.

102 ibid., p. 56.

103 ibid., pp. 74–5.

104 F. M. Martin, *Between the Acts: Community Mental Health Services 1959–1983* (1984), cited in L. K. McLean, N. C. Brady and J. E. McLean 'Reported communication abilities of individuals with severe mental retardation', *American Journal on Mental Retardation*, 100: 580–91 (London: Nuffield Hospital Trust, 1996).

105 Registrar-General, *Statistical Review* (the Seebohm Report).

106 P. Morris, *Put Away: A Sociological Study of Institutions for the Mentally Retarded* (London: Routledge & Kegan Paul, 1969).

107 ibid., p. 315.

108 G. S. Donges, *Policymaking for the Mentally Handicapped* (Aldershot: Gower, 1982), p. 87.

109 H. Smith and H. Brown, 'Inside Out: a Psychodynamic Approach to Normalisation', in H. Brown and H. Smith (eds) *Normalisation: A Reader for the Nineties* (London and New York: Tavistock/Routledge, 1992), p. 93.

110 N. Malin, *Services for People with Learning Disabilities* (London: Routledge, 1995) p. 61.

111 Howe Report, *Report of the Committee of Inquiry into Allegations of Ill Treatment of Patients and Other Regularities at the Ely Hospital, Cardiff,* Cmnd 3975 (London: HMSO, 1969).

112 Watkins Report, *Report of the Farleigh Hospital Committee of Inquiry,* Cmnd 4557 (London: HMSO, 1971).

113 Department of Health & Social Security, *Better Services for the Mentally Handicapped* (London: HMSO, 1971).

114 M. Bayley, *Mental Handicap & Community Care: A Study of Mentally Handicapped People in Sheffield* (London and Boston, MA: Routledge & Kegan Paul, 1973), pp. 9 and 28.

115 Department of Health & Social Security, *Better Services for the Mentally Handicapped* (London: HMSO, 1971).

116 R. Means and R. Smith, *Community Care Policy & Practice* (London: Macmillan, 1994), p. 49.

117 Jay Report, *Committee of Inquiry into Mental Handicap Nursing & Care,* Vol. 1. Cmnd 7468-1 (London: HMSO, 1979).

118 L. Hoyes and L. Harrison, 'An Ordinary Private Life', *Community Care*, 12 February 1987: 20–1.

119 Means and Smith, *Community Care Policy & Practices*, p. 29.

120 Gillian Wagner, *Residential Care: A Positive Choice*, report of the Independent Review of Residential Care, National Institute for Social Work (London: HMSO, 1988), p. 1.

121 ibid. p. 8.

122 ibid.

123 ibid., p. 32.

124 ibid., p. 31.

125 ibid., p. 33.

126 Social Services Committee, *Second Report: Community Care*. House of Commons Paper 13-1, Sessions 1984–5 (London: HMSO, 1985).

127 ibid.

128 Means and Smith, *Community Care Policy & Practice*, p. 50.
129 Audit Commission, *Making a Reality of Community Care* (London: HMSO, 1986).
130 Sir Roy Griffiths, *Community Care: Agenda for Action*, report to the Secretary of State for Social Services (London: HMSO, 1988), p. vi.
131 ibid., p. 5.
132 ibid., p. 6.
133 ibid., p. 56.
134 ibid., p. 219.
135 Department of Health, *Caring for People: Community Care in the Next Decade and Beyond* (London: HMSO, 1989), p. 22.
136 ibid., p. 17.

2   The case for citizenship

RIGHTS, CITIZENSHIP AND SOCIAL POLICY

The most fundamental institution in British society concerned with rights and citizenship is the law itself. The law provides a structure for society involving the constitution, charters of rights and the juridical system. Social policy provides another powerful structure through which rights and citizenship are established and accessed, but the boundaries of rights and citizenship have become blurred when legal attempts have been made at defining the rights of people with learning disabilities, and more particularly those with profound disabilities. Different disabled people need different forms of help if they are to achieve equal capacity. Stainton (1994)[137] believes that the challenge for social policy is to create a method by which individuals can articulate their choices and needs, enabling the state to meet realistic claims in a way that does not take away individual autonomy. He suggests that social policy must aim to create a means for dialogue between the individual, his or her claims and the state. From the late 1970s, the Labour government attempted to address this question by introducing the social inclusion debate, and establishing a means of consumer participation in service planning. In the case of people with learning disabilities, consumer participation was first suggested as a tool for change with the All Wales Strategy,[138] but the initial problem with the idea of consumer participation was that, with a limited number of exceptions, it rarely meant *consumer power*. Critics remind us that since the idea of consumer participation first began, many service users involved in service planning have said they felt disregarded and held back by a lack of knowledge. Others spoke about the process as simply a 'tokenistic' exercise, with poor communication and a lack of understanding about what 'consumerism' actually means. Within this setting there is a growing concern among some professionals about the increasing expectation, on the part of the service users, of becoming 'pseudo-professionals' in the planning process.[139] Croft and Beresford (1989) highlight the problem by suggesting:

> . . . user groups are increasingly conscious of the problem of being
> sucked into the operational and organisational detail of agencies, when
> what they actually want is more control over their own lives and their
> dealings with them.'[140]

The ideological concept of consumerism and choice brought with it a
change in direction for services planning. However, while the language may
have changed, the reality has not; the 'client', for example, as customer, still
has to accept what is on offer, in terms of services, and in this sense consumer participation is not a rights-based system. A conflict inherent in the
process, is the fact that ultimately defining what the person needs remains
solely in the hands of the care manager as assessor, provider and budget
holder. The reality is that the care manager must work within a limited
budget, and can buy only what can be afforded. Stainton refers to this as
structural paternalism and believes the result at best is often inadequate
services and at worst none at all:

> There are few structural means for the person to influence the nature of
> the services, except, as often was the case, to organise their own alter-
> natives. We can call this "structural paternalism" in that no specific
> person is dictating what is in your best interest, rather it is the structure
> which inherently makes this determination.[141]

A QUESTION OF CHOICE AND FREE WILL

The new liberalism brought about through Thatcherism was a place where
the individual expressed choice in the market. The purpose of the marketisation of services was intended to introduce choice by redirecting or eliminating the state monopoly on service provision. And in much of the
literature, as well as government documents published in this area in the
past two decades, elements of these positions may be found. There is no
hint here of the determinism evident elsewhere in social work theory, even
though growing importance is attached to behaviourist approaches especially regarding challenging behaviour. The emphasis on choice for people
with learning disabilities comes from a number of sources including the disability movement advocating autonomy through choice and release of
dependency on the care system. In the context of Thatcherism, however,
choice is amplified as a virtue of services not liberalism; that is to say, our
identity is expressed through the market. An interesting question asks: *Why
has choice acquired such prominence in the context of service provision in
the field of learning disability?*

In social work generally, free will, the freedom to choose, has been
seen to be at odds with much social work theory on which social work
draws, such as the emphasis on determinist theories associated with

psychoanalysis and behaviourism. In the context of policies for people with learning disabilities there appears to be little attempt to relate the question of choice to this philosophical debate, and there is a tension that is reflected in a long-standing tradition within philosophy.

In ancient Greece the idea of fate seemed to prelude any possibility of experiencing autonomy in the way we live our lives. The notion of *'Moria'* or fate, which is present in ancient Greek literature, is a belief that all our actions are pre-ordained. Our behaviour is the working-out of our destiny. This implies that people do not have any control, choice or free will to shape their own histories.

Christian theologians have also debated the question for centuries. Eileen Munro (1988) tells us:

> They argued that if God, being omniscient, knows everything that has or will happen, then all our future actions are already fixed; the results of our apparently free deliberations are already known to God. Nowadays the success of the natural sciences in developing causal explanations is the major source of doubt over the existence of free will.[142]

The freedom of the will is denied by the determinists and the fatalists, who in one way or another hold that the will is necessitated either from within or from without. Theological determinism denies the freedom of the will, because when God moves the will He determines its act in such a way that there can be no free choice. Fatalism, like theological determinism, holds that everything happens of necessity, is decided by fate.

There are three strands to the discourse: (1) libertarianism: that is to say, we have free will: our actions are not pre-ordained; (2) hard determinism: any sense of free will we have is an illusion because our lives are determined for us; (3) compatibilism: our concepts of determinism and freedom can be reconciled. The compatibilist position has been associated with many writers throughout the ages including Thomas Hobbes (1588–1679) in *Leviathan* (1651: Chapter 21) and *Elements of Law*,[143] John Stuart Mill (1867),[144] A. J. Ayer (1976),[145] and D. Dennett (1984).[146] These authors challenge the argument that:

> When we say we made a free choice we mean that we could have done something else in exactly the same circumstances. We feel free, they suggest, when our own wishes and feelings influence what we do as opposed to times when our movements are wholly caused by outside factors.[147]

These critics suggest that we exercise free will when our actions are influenced by our wishes and feelings, in contrast to those which are caused by external factors. It is an explanation that satisfies neither determinists, who regard this concept of freedom as illusionary, nor libertarians, for whom none of our actions are determined. Libertarians suggest that there is an 'I' within every individual that can reason and make free choices, choosing one of several options. However, some common agreement can be found between libertarians, compatibilists and hard determinists on the question of predictability. They accept that some predication is possible because our behaviour is controlled by regulations. Dennett (1984) believes that human rationality adds a significant and complicated dimension to prediction, because human beings actively appraise experiences, examine information rationally and evaluate responses. We process information in a highly personal manner and our use and evaluation of information enable us to make our choices.[148]

Existentialism deals with the philosophy of individual existence, freedom and choice, but because of the diversity of positions taken within existentialism, it is impossible to define the term precisely. The nearest definition would be: *'the philosophy of the existence of the individual as a free and self-determining agent'*.[149]

A primary theme emerging from existentialist writing is that of choice. Existentialists hold the belief that human beings do not have a 'fixed' nature as do animals and plants, but that each human being makes choices. The 20th-century French philosopher Jean-Paul Sartre proposed that choice is central to human existence and, therefore, inevitably inescapable. Even the act of refusing to choose is of itself a choice. Choice carries with it commitment and responsibility. When a person chooses a course of action, she or he accepts the risk and responsibility that goes with that choice. Sartre believed that the acceptance of personal responsibility is a main value in life, and this position is reflected throughout his plays and novels.[150] Sartre used the word *'anguish'* for the recognition of the total freedom of choice that confronts each individual at every moment.[151] His work is intrinsically atheistic and pessimistic and his philosophy declared that human life requires a rational basis while at the same time it is a 'futile passion'. Nevertheless his work reflects and celebrates the human condition as one of freedom, choice and responsibility.

Critics point out the striking tension that exists between social work professionals and scientific theories. Professionals, for example, see their clients as individuals with free will and attempt to help and understand them by means of empathy and imagination. Scientists in contrast are depicted as strict behaviourists investigating exclusively behaviour while ignoring the complexities of the mental process at work in human beings. The important difference between the approaches of science and those of the professionals is not in the way they attempt to create theories, but in how ideas can be tested. Science offers methods for testing theories empirically, which, scientists say, are more reliable than relying on intuition and empathy alone.

Freedom of choice is about not only having a range of options to choose from, but also having the capacity to make choices. To make a choice implies a certain level of rationality, cognitive understanding and mental ability. Reacting to external stimuli or to instinct cannot be said to be making an active well-informed choice. To have choice suggests autonomy and, in its broadest sense, autonomy can be defined as the capacity of the individual to formulate and act on plans and purposes that are self-determined.[152] The literature on autonomy frequently debates the importance of free will and suggests that free will is characteristically unique to human beings. Individuals act according to purpose not merely out of instinct. Choice, therefore, is reflective of our value base, and acts as an expression of our plans and purposes: what we choose to do or be from a range of options.

Philosophers explore the connection between the idea of rationality and the relationship to rights and choices. Most have chosen to focus on the 'norm' – that is to say, everyday life – and so avoid the complex problems surrounding those outside the norm.[153] Others such as Stainton (1994) argue that even when the individual lacks certain 'rational capabilities', there continues to be a need to respect the basic wishes and choices individuals make. If there is difficulty in expressing choices, because of communication or cognitive impairment, then an 'approximation' must be attempted, on the basis of an agreement of the primary good of the person, which will help to ensure that the rights of the individual are valued regardless of rational capacity or communication ability.[154] With such a theory, however, inevitable questions follow about the subjective nature of choice, rights and communication. What of individuals who lack the skills necessary to communicate or express choice or who make choices which appear to be inappropriate? There is always the danger that it may be argued that because an individual lacks the ability to communicate, he or she also lacks the basic human right of choice. It should never be the case that a person can only possess human rights where capacity, understanding and communication can be easily understood and demonstrated: most people within the normal range of understanding, make inappropriate choices from time to time.

The notion of choice and autonomy is associated with the philosophy of *free will* defined in philosophical and psychological terms as the ability to choose among alternative courses of action and to act on the choice made. Choice has been referred to as *'willed behaviour'* which is in stark contrast to behaviour stemming from instinct, impulse, reflex or habit. The German philosopher Arthur Schopenhauer suggested the will dominated every aspect of an individual's personality, knowledge, feelings and direction in life.

Modernity tends to regard the will as having a more pragmatic function: an aspect or quality of behaviour, rather than a separate faculty. It is the whole individual who wills. Present-day psychology argues that this process has distinct stages:

(1) the fixed attention on relatively distant goals and relatively abstract standards and principles of conduct;
(2) the weighing of alternative courses of action and the taking of deliberate action that seems best calculated to serve specific goals and principles;
(3) the inhibition of impulses and habits that might distract attention from, or otherwise conflict with, a goal or principle;
(4) perseverance against obstacles and frustrations in pursuit of goals or adherence to principles.[155]

Claire had been a carer to Marion for eight years at the time she was interviewed for this study. The type of life Marion wishes to lead highlights the difficulties of capacity, understanding, rights and choice. Claire speaks about her experience:

> We have a young woman, Marion, who has been placed on a permanent basis with us now by social services for quite a few years now. In fact, we first had her to stay as a child, placed by the Children and Families section. Marion has extreme periods of violent behaviour where she smashes her room up. She smashed the bed up last week, the pictures on the wall and most other items in her room. Marion wants to become a nun. She works at St Joseph's Centre with nuns and I think working there has given her a real sense of importance. The Bishop is a very kind man who spoke to us recently and said she needs to have an understanding of the choice she is making. Personally I think she gets fulfilment from working with nuns, they keep me informed about things that are happening at the centre. Choice is something that has to be negotiated in all our lives; the choice to get pregnant without support. The choice not to wash ourselves or have clean clothes.'

This example raises the question about rationality and how rationality can be measured. It cannot be measured in terms of something that is singular and fixed; for example, our approach to a certain course of action may be deemed rational, in one sense or set of circumstances, but not in another. From here the focus shifts to an investigation of boundaries of incompetence in the lives of others. It has been argued that one reason which may justify such interference is because the person is incompetent to make choices.

INCOMPETENCE

Incompetence is generally defined under two headings: *temporary*, as in the case of mental illness; or more *permanent*, such as the state of learning disabilities. However, Stainton (1994) observes:

> One of the problems in trying to sort out the role of incompetence . . .
> is that people rarely exhibit total incompetence, or put another way,
> rarely lack autonomy in all areas of judgement.[156]

According to Murphy in his work 'Incompetence and Paternalism'
(1979)[157] incompetence may arise through:

- ignorance: a lack of sufficient information to make an informed and
  reasonable choice;
- compulsion: where the individual lacks the ability to resist a given
  choice;
- lack of reason: an inability to make a rational choice.

Murphy identifies what he terms basic sub-groups as 'non-rational persons' offering as an example people deemed irrational or unconscious such
as those in a comatose state. A further state of incompetence, not mentioned by Murphy, is incompetence related to expression. An example of
this would be an individual who is inarticulate and unable to communicate choice in a manner that is easily identified and understood with the
added complication of interpretation. This raises the question: *How is it
possible to know if the expression of choice is being fully comprehended?*
A way of understanding this, through a comparison, is to imagine being
on holiday in a foreign country where one cannot understand what is
being said nor enter into a dialogue because one cannot communicate or
express oneself.

Wilkener (1979)[158] believes there is no such thing as a fixed level of intelligence that can be regarded as 'normal'. He argues mental capacity ought to
be seen, not as a matter of intellect, but of competence in terms of the intellect's power to meet a challenge.[159] Incapacity, therefore, can be said to be
related to an inability to make certain choices or carry out certain tasks without causing serious risk to self or others. Such a statement inevitably carries
with it underlying tensions about the value society places on disabled people,
and on particular groups such as the profoundly disabled.

SUBSTITUTE DECISION-MAKING

The aim of substitute decision-making is to protect and enhance the autonomy and quality of life for the individual on whose behalf decisions are
being made. This basically means adopting an *Interpretative Role,* and is
particularly relevant where people have difficulty articulating their needs.
Stainton (1997) suggests two formats for the decision-making process. First,
he speaks about *Substitute Judgement,* describing this as a person attempting to make decisions on behalf of the individual deemed incompetent, that
she or he would have made given the capability, and second, *the Best*

Interests Standard which aims to choose that which any rational person would choose.[160]

For the purpose of promoting personal autonomy, Stainton suggests that substitute judgement is the most important and logical path, but the difficulty is who should take on the responsibility of proxy decision-making, and who is best suited to interpret the choices made. What needs to be considered is the relationship between the two. Parents are the primary example to illustrate this point, making decisions on behalf of their children. This is not to deny the importance of respecting even minimal capacity or extremely limited competencies to make choices, and intervention should not restrict action or choice and must itself be justified. Intervention, by professionals, if not monitored can curtail most if not all autonomous actions as may be seen clearly in the examples of forcible sterilisation policies.

FROM PATERNALISM TO PROTECTION

Undoubtedly the principles of autonomy versus paternalism provided a good reason for closing the large institutions and enabling wide-ranging rights of individuals to be protected. Assisting and respecting the choices made by former patients about where and how they wanted to live was one of the most important of these rights. The ideological goal was to maximise choice through autonomy. Critics[161] argue that because there has been such a long and established tradition of paternalistic service provision, the pendulum began to swing too far in the opposite direction. They point to the fact that those who wished to remain in the institution, where they had lived for most of their adult lives, were not allowed to do so. Paternalism has come to mean something inappropriate, something that demeans the individual instead of something that is necessary to enhance the quality of their life. Bicknell (1992) demonstrates the danger if paternalism is abandoned for people who need it as a counterbalance to the objectives of independence and ordinary life:

> Sarah has Down's Syndrome and lives in a group home. She is 23 years old and comes from a loving and caring family. In the house she has been encouraged to make her own decisions, and has abandoned her slimming diet and her daily bath. She is now grotesquely obese and smells and her hair is rarely washed. She seems unhappy but cannot say why. Her parents are distraught because they feel she needs more supervision and direction and are considering having her home again to live.[162]

This example highlights the need for a balance to be met. There is a difference between keeping a person childlike, and giving her or him the dignified help that many people with learning disabilities need to achieve a realistic sense of autonomy. While this may mean involving the individual, the parent and the professional in taking risks, it has to be done within the boundaries of common sense taking account of the fact that the person has a *'learning'* disability. Part of the role for a number of professionals is to help their users through practical teaching, such as in the case of keyworkers. In the case of Sarah the professionals seriously neglected their duties and responsibilities towards her. Sarah was clearly unhappy and obesity has serious health implications which the staff did nothing to tackle. In many cases professionals seek to justify such actions by arguing that priority must be given to the choice of the individual, while parents are criticised for being overprotective. The emphasis is on the importance of allowing the person to take risks, which often results in conflict between the parents and professionals. One solution is for parents and professionals to work together to create a framework within which people can experience greater autonomy in relative safety and avoid situations like Sarah's. Bicknell (1992) continues by drawing attention to the complex nature of choice:

> It is easy to offer choices to those who have never learnt to make them, to offer difficult ones to those who can only manage simple choices, and to offer none at all when it is quicker and more expedient for someone else to make the decision.[163]

CONSENT, CAPACITY AND THE LAW

In many ways the real framework within which we live our lives reflects tensions between a general assumption about the equality people have in relation to freedom and choice, while excluding certain categories of people from any possibility of exercising this freedom. The current legal position states that as citizens we have an inherent right to self-determination and the right to autonomy. Common law works on the assumption that every citizen has 'competency', that is to say, each individual is competent to make decisions and consequently is responsible for those decisions unless proven otherwise.[164] The problem for people with learning disabilities is that assumptions about their inability to make valid choices have often already been made. Claire highlights this difficulty:

> 'Marion doesn't even have the choice to have her own bank account: everything seems to end up in a court of law these days. With a bank account, the need from the social workers' point of view is for a Court of Protection order, they may ease up on that one though with the new bill that is going through just now.[165] In law nobody has a choice, look at the case about the woman with learning difficulties whose mother wants her sterilised. That's gone to court for the court to make the choice not her.'[166]

There are various ways oppression continues to operate; for example, many organisations will not accept people with learning disabilities as trustees. Not accepting people with learning disabilities as trustees is based, not on any test of individual capacity, but on a blanket assumption of incapacity, with added weight given to the argument that the position of trustee is one of considerable responsibility. Having incapacity in one area of an individual's life does not necessarily mean having incapacity for self-determination in all areas of life. A dangerous precedent can be set by professionals who go down the road of limiting opportunities for choice, or excluding service users from participation based on such assumptions. However, attempts are being made to change this. The White Paper *Valuing People* (2001)[167] makes clear the government's commitment to people with learning disabilities in support of their legal and civil rights. It states:

> The Government is committed to enforceable civil rights for disabled people in order to eradicate discrimination in society. People with learning disabilities have the right to a decent education, to grow up to vote, to marry and have a family, and to express their opinions, with help and support to do so where necessary . . . All public services will treat people with learning disabilities as individuals with respect for their dignity, and challenge discrimination on all grounds including disability. People with learning disabilities will also receive the full protection of the law where necessary.[168]

COMMUNITY AND EMPOWERMENT

This attempt at creating a framework within which civil rights might be guaranteed seems to go some way towards giving some meaning to, and providing a basis for, the development of empowerment. Along with '*community care*', '*user empowerment*' became a theme for the 1990s; however, defining exactly what the term 'empowerment' means remains a problem. Contributors to the debate, such as the disability movement, and advocates of the ordinary life approach highlight the difficulties the concept of empowerment creates. Similar problems arise when trying to define 'Community'. The term 'community care' has become firmly established in the English language, but it continues to be a vague sentiment with many meanings and unhelpful interpretations, and loaded with confusion. Originally, the term came into being as a way of denoting non-institutional care. Care *in* the community as opposed to care *by* the community reflects the different ways 'community' can be interpreted. The first of these currently constitutes the idea of community, while the latter is seen as the role the community takes. Bulmer (1987) argues that these concepts

... rest on fallacious common-sense assumptions which are wrongly presented by policy makers as sociological truths. As a result there is a vacuum at the heart of care policy, which is likely to lead to ineffective or deteriorating provision of services.[169]

To illustrate the problem in the context of learning disabilities, it is often argued that a goal for policy makers should be to enable people with learning disabilities to participate in the building of the community as equal citizens. This call for equality is reflected in the more recent literature that focuses on social inclusion, rejecting established service provision as being the suitable answer. A prominent contributor to the discourse is the American writer John McKnight. McKnight began to gain influence in Britain during the early 1990s, with his vision of community as one that is based on an anti-professional stance and against the 'disabling' service systems. This was also Wolfensberger's point of view. McKnight argues that if people with learning disabilities are to be integrated successfully into the community, then it must be the responsibility of the community to support them. McKnight's *Community Vision* sees the community as a place where all contribute their gifts equally. Community needs to become the political defender of the rights of labelled people to be free.[170] However, the reality of integrating people with learning disabilities into society on equal terms is one that remains highly questionable, divorced from everyday life. The struggle to participate in community is often felt as an impossible task to achieve for many. 'A meeting in McDonalds' is a moving account of one mother's experience of community with her disabled daughter Kate. It helps us to understand the problem of an individualised approach and community integration:

A Meeting in McDonalds[171]

Kate and I are parched. It's early, the air is hot and dry. Kate and I need a drink . . . I've got a towel . . . She's telling me, in her own language, that she's dying of thirst. I see her mouth is dry . . . I know we'll pass a McDonald's. "Well, it's still early," I reassure myself, "there won't be many people in." We've not been in for ages. We've not been out together for ages! Over the past two or three months we've been through a lot . . . They have all taken their toll on my courage and stamina. This morning I feel brittle and extremely vulnerable. I couldn't stand all the stares and silence. Those looks, that people wear when they're trying to work out what's wrong with my beautiful daughter. The look of pity washing over some of their faces, the blank expression which covers like a mask, but worst of all are the demonstrations of disgust and loathing.

Back at my seat I concentrate on giving Kate the milkshake. She just loves McDonald's milkshakes. "Drink," I say, touching Kate's bottom lip gently with the large beaker, warning her something was coming. I raise the cup to her beautiful pink perfect lips so that a few thick creamy brown drops stain her open mouth. Her tongue takes it, she swallows, there's a slight pause and she opens her mouth wide, just like a baby song thrush wanting more. I tentatively look around, to see whether they are still looking. Everyone is busy eating and chatting. I can now relax and let my defensives fall. I start to enjoy myself. I just love it when Kate enjoys things and she is certainly enjoying the milkshake.

"Amy, Amy come back here, your chips are getting cold," shouts a high-pitched female voice with just a hint of panic . . . Too late! Amy, a two-and-a-half-year-old, has spotted Kate's giant pushchair and is darting towards it. She has a few French Fries grasped tightly. She comes to investigate. She's never seen such a big girl sitting in a pushchair before. I smile. Amy looks at Kate, a puzzled stare. Amy is quiet. Kate can't hear Amy, so doesn't realise that she is near. Amy doesn't understand why Kate hasn't acknowledged her presence . . . I eventually stutter, "Hello Amy, this is Kate."

"Amy come here at once, your chips are getting cold." Her Mum is looking embarrassed . . . I want to explain. I want her to understand. To accept. Amy is running to her Mum. She is pointing to Kate. Her mother and I stare the same dumb understanding. I smile inanely. It's supposed to tell her mother it's OK.

"Sit down and eat your chips," her Mum is telling her. Amy obeys.

She turns around once more, her red-ringed mouth open, as if about to ask those important questions. I smile. I don't know what else to do . . . I'm trying to hide the hurt. I'm looking into Kate's deep blue unseeing eyes. I look deeper and deeper as if I'm trying to find the answers or the ways to help me and Kate feel that we belong to the community that we were born into.

I'm looking at her face and I just wonder. Her mouth is ringed with brown, she is content and satisfied. I push the hurt away. I say, "My goodness, you're enjoying the milkshake." She opens her mouth wide for more.

It is an experience of community which seems to mock the idea not only of community but also empowerment, and highlights the importance of formal service provision in guaranteeing a reasonable experience of life for people with learning disabilities. However, defining exactly what the term 'empowerment' means remains a problem. The Oxford Dictionary defines it as 'Authorise, enable, (person to do)'. Contributors to the debate, such as the disability movement, and advocates of the ordinary life approach, highlight the difficulties the concept of empowerment creates. Empowerment is essentially about 'power' and it attempts to enable users to have more control over their lives.

ADVOCACY AND EMPOWERMENT

Initially, service users were excluded from many areas of planning including 'steering groups' set up to examine the best ways of providing community-based services. Since that time increased importance has been attached to involving users in the planning of their social services, and a significant development during the past decade, has been the growth of the advocacy movement. The advocacy organisation People First, for example, has a full-time office in London offering work and training to people with learning disabilities. People First offers user perspectives on services through discussion groups, gives one-to-one interviews and publishes on a wide range of topics.[172] Many of its users have ideas and thoughts about the services they receive, and about the lack of services too, and local authorities have been keen to canvass these views. However, there remains the dilemma that if a user is articulate she or he runs the risk of being seen as unrepresentative of the majority of people with learning disabilities, but if the user is not articulate the problem is for him or her to represent themselves or be represented in such a way as to have any real influence over change. This is where the advocate steps in and the Disabled Persons Act 1986 (Sections 1–3)[173] refers to advocates and independent representatives, outlining the scope that exists. However, the Conservative government chose not to implement Sections 1–3, because of the cost implications.

Advocacy in recent years has taken on a variety of different meanings. Within learning disabilities it has mostly come to mean informal personal support that includes, in broad terms, family, friends and workers who act independently of social service professionals. The role of the advocate, in part, has been developed in response to the growing emphasis on resource constraints. Advocates often feel outside 'the system' and it is not unusual for them to report a sense of hostility from social service professionals. Advocates say this has dramatically increased with the change and growth of emphasis on the person with front-line responsibility for resource constraints.[174] Many, although not all, professionals see advocates as impeding the decision-making process by taking up valuable time which could be better used in the planning and delivering of services.

Jacinta was a social worker who had worked in the learning disabilities section for 25 years. When she was interviewed for this study it was clear that she saw advocates as trouble-makers who did not appreciate her work, and indeed set out to undermine it:

> 'Advocates – well it's all very difficult for social workers. Most don't understand our users. We have taken the referral and looked at how we are going to try to meet the users' needs. I honestly don't know why there's a lack of communication between us and the advocates. I had a situation with one of them recently where I felt I was communicating the problems very clearly, and I thought they understood. Things like the politics behind the situation, the dilemmas, you know funding that sort of thing. This is what I'm talking about, but they pitted the users against me in a way that I as a care manager simply wouldn't do. You know I genuinely think they see their role as trouble shooters. I don't think I'd push my views to such an extent and risk the whole service, the continuity. If you take that approach I don't think you ever reach the end of the task that you are working towards. Advocates should explain more about the process instead of acting as trouble shooters as I see it.'

In contrast to Jacinta's views, Ismail, a commissioning manager in the same department, adopted a much more positive approach to advocates and saw them as a valuable resource:

> 'Communication is a difficult area especially with users who have profound problems. Advocates usually have a useful overview, I mean they know people in different settings and situations. They expect more feedback for their user from us. My experience with advocates is that they have a really sound attitude, no axe to grind against the staff, and don't have the pre-conceptions that some of our managers do.'

Meaningful participation by service users, their families and advocates is vastly limited because, at the present time, neither families nor advocates have any real power over the decision-making process.[175] Yet most local authorities promote their services as *rights-based systems*, with *social inclusion,* and *valuing diversity.* They are required to promote central government policy, directives and guidance on legislation and must work within its limitations. Many organisations argue the need to formally recognise the status of advocacy within the decision-making process, and attempts have recently been made to move more towards a formalisation of advocacy born out of pressure brought from families and friends. One of the most widely known in this country is *Citizen Advocacy.* Citizen advocates tell us that their legitimacy is to be found in their primary role as providing advocacy to disabled people over a long period, where the relationship and support grow mutually.[176] They aim to develop a personal bond and commitment with the individual, and citizen advocates seek to build a relationship with disadvantaged individuals. Most advocates are not employed, but work on a voluntary basis with training and support given by the organisations to which they have offered their services. Some other forms of advocacy include *Corporate Advocacy*, which has been developed over the past few years, and is a type of advocacy that is applied to groups advocating for changes to social policy. Another readily recognisable, and well-known, form of advocacy, is that of self-advocacy. Self-advocacy is a movement formed by groups or individuals who have experienced disadvantage. In this country People First is the most commonly associated organisation currently involved in self-advocacy for people with learning disabilities. People First has two main objectives:

(1) to promote and support self-advocacy through peer support, informing people of their rights, and advocacy skills acquisition;
(2) group advocacy on issues of concern to the members.[177]

Arguably, self-advocacy is useful only to those with a high level of communication. A more recent development has been a rise in support groups for families. These groups enable families to make their position as advocates a powerful one, and it has been known for them to act as corporate advocates also. Advocacy performs the vital function of ensuring support to individuals to communicate their preferences in a rights-based system. It further acts as a method for keeping the system in check ensuring the user's rights and choices are respected.

Wolfensberger is one of the main critics of the advocacy movement, but his criticism is aimed not so much at the role of advocacy as such, but at its employment within organisations providing services, and he points to the potential conflict. He believes advocates should be independent from the statutory body, and argues organisations involved in advocacy must not be part of the structure relating to non-advocacy service provision. Many professionals interviewed for this study agreed with Wolfensberger. Kunle, for example, is a senior manager who highlights an important potential danger that can arise when the boundaries are blurred:

'Professionals are employed by social services and therefore they are bound by the terms and conditions of their employment. They are restricted to what they can say and do. I'm not suggesting that professionals don't advocate on behalf of their user, of course they are doing that all the time, it is part of their role. The easiest example I can give is where they are providing a residential or daycare service to people. Part of this role is to advocate for people, but they are bound within the organisation. They may also have their own vested interest, career progression for example, which is all well and good and how it should be for staff who want to get on. What I am saying is if they fail the user they can't advocate against themselves, do you get what I mean? An advocate theoretically shouldn't have a vested interest whatsoever. They shouldn't be related to the person: they shouldn't be employed by an organisation that provides the service the person is in receipt of, but should be there purely to speak on behalf of that individual and have their best interests at heart. There are several different sorts of advocate which to my mind makes things complicated, especially for users and their families. There are some advocates where the advocate just helps the person if they want to make a complaint, then others who help when some legal process needs sorting, and others who don't want to get too involved. Some advocates want to become a daily voice for the service user, I find that particularly difficult. For me an advocate is someone who is multi-faceted in the sense that they are there to help the person hold their providers accountable. They support the person with learning difficulties to reach their goals and have a voice, maintaining their rights and putting forward the person's opinions. I think there are real issues about communication tied up in all this, it becomes very complicated when users don't communicate in conventional ways. More needs to be done about advocacy; it shouldn't be the case anyone can walk in from the street and be a person's advocate. But it must be independent from social services staff.'

Currently advocacy organisations rely on the support of local authority funding and, therefore are not truly independent bodies. Thomas is a strategic planning manager who believes advocates need to challenge professionals more, but in order for them to be in a position to do this in an effective way, he argues, they must be completely independently funded which would help to strengthen their position. He said:

'I think there are many kinds of advocate. I think our care managers have to advocate in one way. By that I mean they have to keep in mind that they are employed by the department, and they therefore have certain responsibilities and loyalties towards the organisation. They must retain a certain degree of advocacy for their client otherwise they wouldn't be doing their job, but in no way can that be full-blown advocacy by virtue of the way they work. I think the type of advocacy most people think about is one that is completely independent of the statutory organisation. They owe nothing to anyone except the person with learning difficulties, and that can be a most powerful form of advocacy. The power of that kind of advocate is only limited when inhibited by who's funding that advocate then you get a bit of a conflict. I'm trying to think of a good recent example I can offer that happened in this department. Yes, I funded a women's group and these women are most powerful advocates, but they'd be more powerful if when they came to me to complain about whatever was going on, that I wasn't the one funding them. If there was independent funding it would be much better. In this borough at present there is no completely and independently funded advocacy service for people with learning difficulties. The best we have achieved is a limited amount of distributed funding mostly through partnership working with health. Complete independence and separate funding would enable them as a group to be much stronger and I do approve of that. We need to be challenged all the time and we're not challenged enough. At the present time there are 600 people with a learning difficulty in this borough and perhaps a dozen of them have advocates if that.'

The White Paper *Valuing People* is innovatory in terms of the importance it sees advocacy playing in the lives and support networks for people with learning disabilities, '. . . which is brilliant', comments Jean Collins of Values into Action, '. . . there is a lot about advocacy in the paper, but are they really going to give precedence to what the person with a learning difficulty actually says? If the White Paper is going to make a difference to the lives of people with learning difficulties it has to put their choices first.'[178]

Rupert Erdley is the only full-time advocate working in the borough investigated by this study. He manages a large advocacy organisation which spans two central London boroughs, and receives some funding from both. Rupert speaks extensively about his experience of being an advocate in the borough, and how he has been viewed by the professionals. He makes comparisons between the attitudes of the professionals in each of the boroughs. He talks about the relationship between advocacy and a number of related themes including communication, choice, inclusion, and independence. Rupert began by giving a general explanation of citizen advocacy in the context of communication difficulties, illustrating some of the points made earlier in this discussion:

'If you look at something like Best Value what does it tell us for the lives of people with learning disabilities? It tells us you need to be articulate, able-bodied and a political person. Most users don't understand basic questions – Where do you live? If asked outright questions – Do you like your home? – they will answer yes. If you take time and do it in a story form this works very well and the results can be good. One young man was frustrated, we didn't know why, but we knew him well enough to tell by his behaviour. With time and through using the story method he told us "I never get to choose who I live with."

The idea of communication and social inclusion works differently in this borough. There was a day organised when the joint commissioning manager or some such senior person was coming to the day centre. The

day was organised with no agenda. Service users turned up not knowing why they were there. They were bombarded with questions they
didn't understand. About the only thing the day achieved was that users
did not want their staff to change. This was a really bad way of going
about consultation. The other thing that came out was that users
wanted the independent living scheme to stay. I began by talking about
the most appropriate way to mix the groups to help the people have
some understanding about the abstract ideas. One group was more
articulate than the other, but we also had an art group who couldn't
communicate. They didn't mix the groups up and didn't take on board
what I was trying to tell them.'

Rupert gives an example of the citizen model in action when he feels it is
properly used by the local authority:

'Advocacy is complex, it is easy to become everything for the users. If
advocating, I need to always be aware of the independent position I
am adopting. My role is to be the "voice" for the person. It's about
having a knowledge about someone, what they want from services
and then, if necessary, articulating that need. The person who knows
them best can be in the best position for them. I support a service user
and work with them to help them get what they want. That doesn't
mean to say I have to know them well but it's about working with
them, helping them to make choices. Let me give an example. We had
one man who could not communicate his needs. We knew there was
a problem and questioned whether he wanted to move from the residential unit where he lives to a home of his own? It is incredibly difficult. What we did know was that he wasn't happy in his residential
unit because of his emotions and behaviour displayed this, and we set
about monitoring the situation over a number of months. I thought
about the ways I would explore with him, what triggers his behaviour
making him act in a certain way, keeping in mind this may be the way
he displays choice.

I know a profoundly disabled woman who you would imagine could
never make a choice, but she does with her eyes. How do we know she
is making a choice? The real basis to answering this and the wider
answer about advocacy is knowing the person.

Citizen is about one on one. Taking a year to get to know the person
is about right. We have had people as citizen advocates for five or six
years and it works well, the down-side is when the advocate leaves. I
know I realise myself, whenever I say I'm independent I become more
aware of the bigger picture.

As I said I work for two London social services departments. They
both work in quite different ways. With the other borough the person
I work with in the learning disabilities section has been there for a few

years. I have been here for just over a year now. With that borough part
of the referral process and care plan involves advocacy. They speak
with the individual and see if the person wants an advocate and how
the advocate could be of use. That doesn't happen with the borough we
are talking about today. Without being too cynical, if it suits them to
have a different "voice" then they involve us. For example, there was a
case not that long ago where an elderly man with learning difficulties
was moved from the old people's home where he had lived for many
years. This caused problems for the professionals because they said he
needed to move. The advocate should have been involved before the
person was moved. I would be the "voice" saying he does not want to
move, and supporting that person against what the professionals – purchasers and providers want.'

Rupert continued highlighting the difficulties of rights versus action:

'We get a lot of this sort of thing. What we do is question why they
hadn't been referred before. In this case I could have supported him
in his choice not to move. For people with learning disabilities it's a
question of understanding the choices you are being given.

We are involved at committee level when councillors and officers
meet. We can of course ask questions about service planning but we are
pretty powerless to do anything other than ask questions.

Advocacy I'd say it's not a political movement it's about working
with individuals. An advocate is a "voice" for the user not something
that confronts the system. You can't fight the system because your role
is to be a voice for that individual, do you see what I mean?
Respecting the users' choices is an important part of our independence, even when you know their choices are not in their best interests
you respect them.

My answer to all these issues around choice, independence, communication and the rest is education. There needs to be an educational
process to teach people they can complain. It's OK to complain, but it
is not the role of advocacy to take them down this road.

Those who I see as being let down the most are those living independently, what that really means is without support. They don't need
support workers to help them, their independence deems them a success. One user I know of said, "I want more support, I want more help."
The social worker told him, "You don't need more support." He turned
to Octa to help him and when Octa went around to his flat it was
squalid and infested with cockroaches. Moving people into their own
flat means support, but ironically the more successful your move is seen
to be the less help you need and get. The attitude is one of: we are
pleased with your success so we will pull away all your support. That
results in an isolation that nobody wants. Service users survive because

they can't come down the ladder again. It needs to reach breakdown for that to happen. It's a real problem and what makes it such a real problem is that it's an idealistic aim for the professionals that had to be achieved.'

The future of advocacy

The belief underlying *Valuing People* is that the role of the advocate is a very powerful one that helps to transform the lives of people with learning disabilities, arguing that advocates enable users to make choices and express themselves by playing an active part in service planning, which is both relevant to their needs and responds directly to their choices. Interestingly, the White Paper states: 'This applies to people with profound disabilities and to the less severely disabled,' but no practical suggestions are offered to indicate how this might be done. Both citizen advocacy and self-advocacy are praised in the White Paper for their valuable contribution enabling users to have a voice. At the same time the paper also points to the barriers that have hindered the development of the advocacy movement, which include:

- insecure funding;
- limited support for local groups;
- potential conflicts of interest with statutory agencies who provide funding.[179]

The government proposes establishing a range of independent advocacy services, working with advocacy groups to promote a greater development of citizen advocacy and self-advocacy. To ensure this aim is successful, it has pledged over the next three years to invest £1.3 million.[180]

NORMALISATION

Alongside moves to alter political thinking towards people with learning disabilities and bring about changes to legislation, there emerged the 'ordinary life' movement which called for ordinary life practices for people seen as outside the norm. Influenced by British ideas the *Normalisation Principle* first emerged during the late 1950s and early 1960s in Scandinavia. It began when nurses in the hospitals in Scandinavia attempted to make the environment as normal as possible for the patients. It was not about making the patients themselves normal or taking them out of hospitals, and it was this simple philosophy that laid the foundations of the Ordinary Life Movement, which called for the theory to be turned into practical working social policy. In the 1960s, normalisation gathered such support in Denmark and Sweden, that it succeeded in having a direct impact on policy makers and as a consequence led to people with learning disabilities having their rights enshrined in legislation. Originally, the Normalisation Principles were relatively straightforward: *to make the quality of life the same for disabled people as for non-disabled, based on notions of equality, quality of life and quality of services.*[181] The Swedish pioneer of normalisation, Bengt Nirjie, concluded that the new and radical policies were enabling people with learning disabilities to live their lives as near to everyday normal circumstances and patterns of life as possible. Normalisation, he suggested, did not seek to make the disabled normal, rather it aimed to make their life-conditions normal within the limits of their disability.

During the past couple of decades normalisation has become the most important ideology to influence attitudes and ideas towards people with learning disabilities. Unfortunately, the theory has had many varied interpretations in its development into a sociological theory by Wolfensberger, often leading to confusion. The principles of normalisation are rooted in the Sociology of Deviance and Labelling Theory, but essentially it is concerned with the social role of the individual, exploring ways to bring about changes in attitude towards disability in the hope of eliminating the 'deviant role'.[182] Critics have argued normalisation is unrealistic in nature, and can only work with the most articulate and independent individuals. They view the idea as one that seeks to *humanise, cure* and more importantly make *normal* people with learning disabilities. Stainton (1994) believes that:

> each of these raises serious issues, the most common, and the most germane, is the critique that normalisation imposes externally derived 'norms' onto people, that it creates the 'appearance of normalcy' by forcing conformity.[183]

A further criticism levelled at normalisation is that the emphasis is more concerned with the collective organisation, than the choices of the individual.

Wolfensberger answered his critics by offering an explanation of normalisation and choice as he saw them suggesting:

> . . . first, one pursues a line of persuasion, pedagogy, modelling and other forms of culturally normative social influence to steer a person towards a course of action one desires. Second, one imposes coercion only where one would do so legally in the larger societal context . . . Third, one chooses the least restrictive alternative if one does coerce.[184]

The post-normalisation debate of the late 1970s is one that has increasingly emphasised choice, with John O'Brien being one of its foremost advocates.[185] However, the theory itself remains focused on developing service systems with little thought given as to how best to develop the autonomy of each individual. Therefore, normalisation is paternalistic in essence, offering little to social policy in the sense of establishing a method for social administration based on the rights of the users. From its conception normalisation has lacked a strong theoretical framework within which appropriate policies to improve the immediate quality of life for people with learning disabilities could be developed.

Wolfensberger attempted to create a theoretical and academic base for normalisation during the early 1970s. He 'Americanised' the theory, framing it within a sociological context, defining it as:

> . . . utilisation of means which are as culturally normative as possible, in order to establish and/or maintain personal behaviours and characteristics which are as culturally normative as possible.[186]

In other words, Wolfensberger argued the purpose of normalisation was to prevent and even reverse deviancy which, as a social construction, could be socially redefined. While he argued mostly for changing the individual, he also suggested it was about adopting a positive approach towards differentness, and valuing people rather than adhering to culturally normative practices. This illustrates the ambiguous nature of Wolfensberger's approach to normalisation. The subsequent wider debate asks the question: *What does it mean to be socially valued?* Normalisation emphasises the importance of treating people properly and decently in all aspects of their lives, calling for equality of opportunity in education, housing, leisure and employment and participation.

Supporters of Wolfensberger argue that his thesis *The Principle of Normalization in Human Services,* published in 1972, was instrumental in bringing about a change in policy for people with learning disabilities. Wolfensberger, always a controversial figure, provoked strong reaction among both supporters and critics alike with comments such as '*the world seeks to destroy those it has labelled as disabled*' and '*statutory services are damaging*'. Critics, while acknowledging the contribution he has made, now believe it is time to move away from Wolfensberger's ideological vision of normalisation and turn instead towards a paradigm in which disability is perceived as a cultural entity that exists within a specified set of social conditions.[187]

Wolfensberger's normalisation ideology seems unrealistic in the context of the experiences of many parents. Charlotte Moore is one such parent who, writing in the *Guardian* newspaper, described life with her autistic teenage son. The title of her article 'Mind the Gap' reflects just how far removed her son's experience of adolescence is from that of a normal teenager. She said:

'George has changed. For years, he was "the easy one" all things being relative – but this is no longer so. He has turned 12, and adolescence has begun. Much has been written about autistic children. I'd done little more than vaguely imagine my sons as taller, stronger versions of their present selves.

George displays the symptoms in a simplified, almost abbreviated form. He rejects authority. He is automatically negative, even about things he likes. The phrases George uses are essence of teen spirit. "Don't look at me!" "Don't ask me that!" "I don't want to be clean!" "I want holes in my teeth!" His only exercise is dancing to rock music, played – of course – too loud. He has become more socially aware, for the first time wanting to be part of the crowd. He likes Dido and the Pop Idol he matily refers to as "William", but last night his choice of video was Teletubbies Bedtime. And that's where the differences begin. No normal 12-year-old could watch Teletubbies except in a spirit of irony. Irony doesn't exist for George Kevin Smith. Satire, black humour, a mocking reappraisal of the adult world, its flaws newly revealed to the average teenager . . .. All this is irrelevant to George. So, too, is the youthful idealism that believes the world can be reinvented. For George, the world doesn't exist beyond the limits of his own experience. What other people think or know does not matter. Like a little emperor, he demands that his "friends" be brought into his presence, but he cannot imagine that they have lives that go on when he's not there. His increased sociability is encouraging, but he still has no empathy.

The painful, comic struggle of adolescence, turning children into adults with a coherent social function, exists only in part for George. The emergence of his identity is actually more like that of a three-year-old. His sense of self may never be whole enough to bear the presence of social responsibility. George becomes distressed at talk of growing up. "I won't be a man; I will be a boy!" Anyway why upset him? Perhaps he never will be a man in any sense other than the physical. Perhaps never-never land isn't a bad place to be.'[188]

Yet despite the mismatch between theory and experience a version of normalisation remains a powerful influence, not only on service providers, but also on academics working in the area of learning disabilities. Why this should be is largely attributed to O'Brien, who sought to synthesise what he regarded as the essence of the normalisation theory, beset as it was with internal inconsistencies in a set of principles out of which he devised a set of benchmarks against which policies and practice could be judged and developed. He set out to turn the theory into workable terms of reference, and did this by setting out five broad goals for services to achieve. These five goals have become known as *O'Brien's Five Accomplishments;* they are summarised in the panel.

O'Brien's Five Accomplishments

- *Ensuring Users Are Present in the Community* – by supporting their actual physical presence as ordinary citizens in schools, churches, recreation and work.

- *Ensuring Users Are Supported to Make Choices* – about their lives, encouraging people to understand their situation and the options open to them on everyday issues such as who they want to live with.

- *Ensuring that Users' Competence Is Developed* – by developing their skills in natural community environments to reduce the person's dependency, and develop characteristics that other people value.

- *Enhancing Respect for the User* – by developing and maintaining positive reputations for service users, ensuring choice and development as citizens.

- *Ensuring that Service Users Participate in the Life of the Community* – by supporting people's natural relationship with their families, neighbours and co-workers and, where necessary, widening each individual's network of personal relationships.[189]

In Britain supporters adopted normalisation because they argued it would achieve new ways of looking at and understanding the needs of people with learning disabilities, resulting in integration and full participation in service planning. However, critics like Linda Ward (1992) underlined the theory's serious failings concerning race, gender and equity. She observes the theory has an

> ... apparent inability to encompass the different circumstances, aspirations and values of women, black people, disabled people and carers; its uncomfortable emphasis on change of the devalued individual rather than the society in which they live.[190]

It is important to take account of the political climate in Britain during this era, when the normalisation debate was at its height. The discourse was taking place at a time when the Thatcher government set out to change and redefine a whole range of values, from the machinery of local government itself, to the value for money that local authority services provided. Conservative policies attempted to ensure the death of the collectivist ideology embodied in the welfare state, and instead preached the political philosophy of individualism, independence and most importantly self-reliance. Under the Conservatives collectivism was given a new and negative label, that of 'dependency culture', and it is here that the tension inherent in the normalisation theory becomes evident. Normalisation is ambiguous in nature because it supports the Tory vision of self-reliance with the ordinary life philosophy advocating independence for the user, self-reliance and choice, but depends on collectivist interdependence.

A keyworker interviewed for this study spoke about trying to resolve the conflict between normalisation and her responsibilities as a key-worker towards the service user. This conflict creates a tension between the unfettered individualism required of the user, and that person's dependence on publicly provided resources to achieve it. The commit-ment to choice is unrestricted by any service of culturally determined appropriateness.

> 'It's a whole big thing normalisation and our responsibilities as key-workers towards our users. There's a lot of people I have worked with who have a dual diagnosis, learning disabilities and mental health prob-lems. Supporting them to be normal is difficult because a lot of the time it means taking risks. Look at an example say one of my users wants to put the washing machine on at 4 a.m. I will stop him, it's not normal and there's a conflict for us as workers. It's about communicating what's normal and what's not. I have another user who has put his hand through the front window here in the home. It's my job to stop him and what about the other residents?'

Clearly, the theory fails to take account of the power relations that exist between those providing the services and those seeking services, and a problem for professionals. The King's Fund set about investigating this and produced a document, based on structured workshops, called 'An ordinary life: comprehensive locally based residential services for men-tally handicapped people'.[191] The information in this document was dis-tributed to service providers in local authorities and the voluntary sector. Consequently, these organisations pooled together to develop strategies that would ensure that the normalisation philosophy would have a direct impact on service planning and the quality services offered.

Critics believe there has not been a real shift in power from the profes-sionals to the user, suggesting the agenda continues to remain firmly in the hands of the professionals. Professionals dispute this, arguing that they do not see any problem developing equal relationships between themselves and users, working towards shared values and goals. However, the pres-ent study suggests this is in direct contrast with the experiences of many service users like Sandra. Sandra's experiences provide a good illustration to demonstrate this.

> 'I have asked for a social worker as far as I know I've just got stuck. They keep saying I don't need one and I say I do need one. I have never

had one in my lifetime, and I think it's all a matter to do with allocation. I can't be admitted into the learning difficulties team, because in
my test I gained too many points on my test. I'm more angry about
being left on the back burner, because I don't particularly fit into one
service or the other. I know it would be helpful to have a social worker
or I'll just fall through the net.'

Some service users involved in the present study felt the pressure to conform
to normality was a stressful experience for them, and said they had little
help or support from the professionals. For a few these feelings developed
into more serious mental health problems. Tom is a 39-year-old man with
a learning disability who lives independently. He said:

> 'We define normalisation as people with learning difficulties being
> given the same opportunities as non-disabled people. Do I get what I
> want? Sometimes it feels as if I have to negotiate with the staff,
> because what I want and what agencies give me are two different
> things. It's because there's a breakdown in communications between
> departments. I explain to them my needs, and as such they are very
> low, but I do have problems. I wanted a normal life and to get a job
> you see. I have problems writing things down and phone messages.
> They sent us a tape recorder [*answer phone*] and I could play that
> back at my leisure and that didn't fit my need, because I'd have to
> remember to set up the tape and turn it on. Remembering where I'd
> put it and when you're answering the phone you only have a split sec-
> ond to answer it, but it would add to my stress. I went back to the
> department and said "It's adding to my stress." I did apply for a
> course in book keeping and I told the guy, the salesman, that I'd be
> home after 6 o'clock and I rushed home from work at 5.30 and that
> really stressed me out. I tried to negotiate with this man but he didn't
> listen.'

Jonathan, another service user, spoke about similar feelings caused by
work. For him they also had a serious effect on his mental well-being:

> 'I will hopefully get another job soon. I walked out of a job last year
> and that started my depression, that is, along with other things. I was
> working for an organisation for people with learning difficulties as a
> project manager, but found it hard to cope with the pressure.
> Eventually after six months I told my boss I wanted to leave. Basically
> they wanted me to leave so I went.'

Yet Jonathan and Sandra are at the most able end of the learning disability spectrum. It is not surprising then that even some professionals

approach normalisation with caution. Natalie has been a social worker for 18 years in the learning disabilities department. Her views echoed many of her colleagues:

> 'Normalisation, it's a difficult one. We set up services to meet people's needs and to make life as normal as possible for them. It's about expectations and what people want. I know it's a cliché, but what's normal anyway? There are all sorts of problems about people like O'Brien and his five accomplishments. What about those who are non-verbal and physically dependent on other people. We include them as much as possible, but it is difficult. The theory is fine but the reality is a problem.'

For many managers, how people with learning disabilities presented themselves to the world was important for acceptance as normal; indeed, they more than any other group of professionals interviewed for this study drew attention to this. Padhraig is one such senior manager involved in service planning for learning disabilities in the borough. He said:

> 'Normalisation, there's a lot in here isn't there? I think normalisation tries to ensure that we treat people with learning difficulties in a way that is similar to the way we'd all like to be treated, and there's good reason for that. Primarily people's perception of normality is based on an understanding and acceptance of a certain level of ability to communicate. Many people with learning difficulties have a reduced level of communication that has marginalised them. An example in the past would be the young woman who became pregnant before she was married and was unable to communicate in a meaningful way with people why this had happened, and how it had happened. In those days she would have been deemed to be mad, or incapable because of an inability to express what was going on and, therefore, was locked up. Appearance has certainly played a main role in the past and still continues to be important. Some people with learning difficulties have appearances that are not considered to be within the bounds of normality, and I think that can often lead to rejection and therefore marginalisation. That said, I feel the whole social role valorisation ethos; well if you want my honest opinion, no it would start me off on my untypically politically incorrect soapbox. There has grown up too much jargon around normalisation. I respect it as a concept very much so. I see very little of it in practice: I hear an awful lot of lip-service paid to it, and on a bad day I kind of despair of what people are actually talking about. Then some days I do see small pockets of service where people are striving to value people in small ways.'

Errol, another manager, also spoke about the importance of appearance both in an historical sense and how people with learning disabilities are seen today:

'There are issues about society and laws and what is acceptable in society as normal. Those who find themselves outside the laws are marginalised in various ways. A lot of people with learning difficulties also actually physically look different, odd even, and are immediately identifiable as somebody who is not normal. If people don't know very much about learning difficulties, they assume, because of the way society portrays these people through imagery in films and TV, that those who look odd are bad, mad or dangerous. These are ideas that go hand in hand. A member of the public, for example, who sees someone on the street with a particular physical disability or doing something odd, a particular sort of behaviour that's not recognised as normal, can become quite nervous and frightened of them and reject them saying "I don't really want to be anywhere near them." This is because of fear or a lack of understanding or simply not knowing what to say or how to act towards them. History has played its part too. For a long time people with learning difficulties were shut away in institutions in large groups, and when they eventually appeared in public it was in groups dressed in shabby clothing. Not being seen as normal is a lot to do with presentation.

I understand the term normalisation to mean an attempt on the part of professionals to acknowledge some of these historical wrongs, and minimise any possibility of them happening now in various ways. One way is focusing on the individuals themselves and trying to teach things that make them feel more in tune with society. The choices of the user are naturally central to this process. It is a two-way learning process. I mean it is giving learning difficulties people the means by which they can inform society about who they are. Looking at it like this, the longer-term aim of normalisation has been to integrate people with learning difficulties into society. I'm not making my point 100 per cent clear here. I don't mean it is about focusing on the individual to re-model them in such a way as they are made normal or tailored to fit into society. Normalisation is not about making the person normal, forcing them to be normal. I guess what normalisation boils down to in the end is acceptance.'

There were a number of people with learning disabilities in the borough whose experience reflected the normal everyday patterns of life. Tanya is a young woman with Down's Syndrome who enjoys life with her partner in their own home. Much of her independence was the result of a strong and determined mother, who wanted Tanya to have as normal a life as possible. Tanya describes her feelings:

'There has been a lot of talk in the papers about Down's people not looking normal, and having plastic surgery to alter their looks and make them more normal looking. I feel very strongly that plastic surgery should not be done just for appearance. I have Down's Syndrome and I'm happy the way I am. You can't get rid of my happiness. I have rights too. The right to work if I want, and a decent standard of living, and to speak my own mind. I live here in the flat I grew up in with my partner Peter. I have a carer who comes in once a week to help me run my life and I do all my own shopping and go to the post office. I'm not good with money so my brother, he helps me. We have a joint account and we both sign the book. That helps because I can't spend all the money in my bank account. I also have a cleaner who I pay to come once a week. It's a big flat and it would take me a long time to do it on my own.

When I was born, the doctor said to my mother that I was going to be mentally and physically handicapped for the rest of my life. What a silly thing to say. I'm very lucky because my mother wanted me to be independent. She wanted me to have the same education as everyone else and the same chances. She was told I would have to go to a special school. My mother wasn't having any of it. "Over my dead body," that's what my mother told them. Eventually, I did go to the same school as my brother, but my mother had to fight for it. I left school with three CSEs.

I cried and cried when my mom died in 1990. I had to cope with life on my own then. I was frightened and thought: what do I do now? It was a really big change in my life. After mom died I took over the flat and got a job. I've had three jobs. I was an office junior with the Down's Association, that was for 13 years. Then I worked for Octa. It was office work again and I worked on the computer in the office and did errands. Then I was a development officer with an advocacy organisation and worked there for a year.'

Bianca spoke proudly about the normality of her life and independence. She talked about her job and life with her husband.

'Call me B for short. I work for the Council: I'm a laundry assistant for the elderly. I've been there nearly 15 years. I started 24 November 1986. We've got the next liaison group meeting here at the home, did you know that? I need to make up time for that. I've been coming to the clubs for nearly 30 years from 1972 onwards until now 17 February 2000.

I did have a social worker and a support worker, when I began to live independently, but now I ain't got no one. He used to help with my money bits and helped me understand prices. He used to help me save. I got another savings book now that I use. Me and my husband were married. He goes to this day centre; he's one of my pensioners. We go 50/50 on the rent and council tax.'

In more recent years, the normalisation philosophy has continued to have an important influence on shaping services, and professionals are increasingly sensitive to the fact that service users are making choices for themselves. Normalisation has succeeded in raising an awareness of the historical injustices to people with learning disabilities, but paradoxically it has created a situation whereby professionals need to discover how to empower service users to make choices that will have a positive effect on their future service, while attempting to resolve the conflict of working within budget limitations.[192]

NOTES

137 Timothy Stainton, *Autonomy & Social Policy: With Special Reference to Mental Handicap in Ontairio and Britain* (Aldershot: Ashgate, 1994; Brookfield, VT: Avebury, 1994).
138 Graham Harper, "Consumer-led Service Planning", *Community Living* 1, no. 6 (1988).
139 Morag McGrath, "Consumer Participation in Service Planning – the AWS Experience", *Journal of Social Policy*, 18, part 1 (1989): 83–5.
140 Suzy Croft and Peter Beresford, "User Involvement, Citizenship and Social Policy", *Critical Social Policy*, no. 26 (August 1989): 15–16.
141 Stainton, *Autonomy & Social Policy*, p. 324.
142 E. Munro, *Understanding Social Work: An Empirical Approach* (London: The Athlone Press, 1998), p. 105.
143 Thomas Hobbes, *Leviathan*, (ed.) Michael Oakeshott (Oxford: Blackwell, 1966 edn. [1651]). Thomas Hobbes, *The Elements of Law*, (ed.) Ferdinand Tonnies, 2nd edn. M.M. Goldsmith (London: Simpkin, Marshall, 1969).
144 J.S. Mill, *An Examination of Sir William Hamilton's Philosophy* (London: Longman, 1867).
145 A.J. Ayer, *The Central Question of Philosophy* (Harmondsworth: Penguin Books, 1976).
146 D. Dennett, *Elbow Room* (Oxford: Clarendon Press, 1984).
147 Munro, *Understanding Social Work*, p. 106.
148 ibid., p. 108.
149 *Collins English Dictionary*.
150 Internet: *"Sartre, Jean-Paul"*, http://www.encarta.msn.com
151 Internet: *"Existentialism"*; this is the Existentialism page: http://www.connect.net
152 ibid., p. 33.
153 ibid., p. 92.
154 John Rawls, *A Theory of Justice* (Cambridge, MA: Belknap Press, 1971), pp. 508–9.
155 Internet: *"Will"* (*Philosophy and Psychology*): http://www.encarta.msn.com
156 See: Stainton, *Autonomy & Social Policy*, p. 116; Jefferie G. Murphy, "Incompetence and Paternalism", in his *Retribution, Justice and Therapy* (Dordrecht: Reidel, 1979), pp. 166–74. Donald Van Deveer, *Paternalistic Intervention* (Princeton, NJ: Princeton University Press, 1986), p. 346; Onoro O'Neill, 'Paternalism and Partial Autonomy', *Journal of Medical Ethics*, no. 10 (1984).
157 J.G. Murphy, 'Incompetence', p. 116.

158 D. Wilkener, "Paternalism and the Mildly Retarded", *Philosophy and Public Affairs* 8, no. 4: 391.

159 See: O'Neill, *'Paternalism'*, p. 177.

160 Stainton, p. 123.

161 J. Bicknell, 'Philosophical and ethical issues', in *Seminars in The Psychiatry of Learning Disabilities*, Gaskell RO (ed.) (London: The Royal College of Psychiatrists, 1997).

162 ibid., pp. 195–6.

163 ibid., p. 197.

164 G. Roberts 'Capacity and Empowerment', in P. Ramcharan, G. Roberts, G. Grant and J. Borland (eds), *Empowerment in Everyday Life*. (London: Jessica Kingsley, 1997).

165 The carer is making reference to new laws being introduced under government plans to protect adults with a 'mental incapacity'. The government is producing a report that outlines plans to modernise and clarify the law following consideration of the 4,000 responses to the 1997 consultation paper: *Who Decides?* A new statutory definition of incapacity will be based on 1995 proposals from the Law Commission. Under new legislation, carers will be given "general authority to act reasonably for the personal welfare or healthcare of a mentally incapacitated person". It closes gaps in the system that have meant carers had no legal authority to administer as much as an aspirin to someone with mental incapacity. A new Court of Protection will have the power to make decisions on behalf of mentally incapacitated people; to make declarations about mental incapacity; and to appoint managers to make some decisions (Community Care Magazine: 4–10 November 1999).

166 This refers to the landmark decision to overturn a high court ruling in January 2000, to impose a hysterectomy on a 29-year-old woman with profound learning disabilities. The woman's mother sought court backing for the treatment in a bid to protect her daughter from pregnancy. Mencap's head of campaigns at the time, Richard Kramer, said the judgment was clearly in the best interests of the daughter. He argued that the sterilisation issue raised fundamental moral questions, saying it cannot be in the person's best interests if based on social rather than medical grounds. The mother was worried the daughter would be at risk when she moved into sheltered accommodation. Dame Elizabeth Butler-Sloss, president of the High Court Family Division, said that, while she sympathised with the mother, a hysterectomy would be "out of proportion at this stage, to the problem to be solved". The daughter, she said, had the right not to have drastic surgery unless it is in her best interests. Kramer said of the judgment that "Her rights are paramount". (*Community Care*: 25–31 May 2000.)

167 Department of Health, *Valuing People: A New Strategy for Learning Disability for the 21ˢᵗ Century*. White Paper, Cm 5086 (London: HMSO, 2001).

168 ibid., p. 23.

169 Martin Bulmer. *The Social Basis of Community Care* (London: Unwin Hyman, 1987), p. ix.

170 John McKnight. "Regenerating Community", address to the Search Conference of the Canadian Mental Health Association, Ottawa, 28 November, 1985.

171 Sue Thomas, 'A Meeting in McDonalds', in *Telling Our Own Stories: Reflections on Family Life in a Disabling World*, (eds) Pippa Murray and Jill Penman (Sheffield: Parents with Attitude, 2000), pp. 241–4.

172 L. Ward, 'Equal Citizens: Current Issues for People with Learning Difficulties and Their Allies', in *Values & Visions: Changing Ideas in Services for People with Learning Difficulties*, (eds) T. Philpot and L. Ward (Oxford: Butterworth-Heinemann, 1995).

173 Department of Health, Disabled Persons (Services, Consultation & Representation) Act (1986). HMSO, London.
174 Stainton, *Autonomy & Social Policy*, p. 331.
175 G. Allan Roeher Institute, *The Power to Choose* (North York: G. Allan Roeher Institute, 1989).
176 John O'Brien, *Learning from Citizen Advocacy* (Tucker, Georgia: Georgia Citizen Advocacy Office, 1987). A further discussion can be found in Morag McGrath and S. Humphreys, *The All Wales Community Mental Handicap Team Survey* (Bangor: University College of North Wales, 1988).
177 Bill Worrell, *Advice For Advisors* (Downsview: National People First Project, 1988), pp. 15–18.
178 Internet: *"Let them Speak"* (17-9-2000): http://www.community-care.co.uk
179 'Department of Health,' *Valuing People*, pp. 46–7.
180 ibid., p. 47.
181 A. Alaszewski and H. Roughton, 'The development of Residential Care for Children with Mental Handicap', in A. Alaszewski and B. N. Ong (eds), *Normalisation in Practice: Residential Care for Children with Profound Mental Handicap* (London: Routledge, 1990), p. 22.
182 Wolf Wolfensberger, "A Brief Overview of The Principle of Normalization", in *Normalization, Social Integration and Community Services*, (eds) Robert J. Flynn and Kathleen E. Nitsch (Baltimore, MD: University Park Press, 1980).
183 Stainton, *Autonomy & Social Policy*, p. 315.
184 Wolf Wolfensberger, "The Definition of Normalization: Update, Problems, Disagreements and Misunderstandings", in *Normalization, Social Integration and Community Services*, (eds) by Robert J. Flynn and Kathleen E. Nitsch (Baltimore, MD: University Park Press, 1980), p. 110.
185 John O'Brien and Connie Lyle, *Introducing Framework for Accomplishment* (Lithonia, Georgia: Responsive Systems Associates, 1986).
186 Wolf Wolfensberger, *The Principles of Normalization in Human Services*, (Toronto: National Institute on Mental Retardation, 1972), p. 28.
187 M. Oliver, *The Politics of Disablement* (London: Macmillan, 1990).
188 Charlotte Moore, "Mind the Gap", *Guardian*, 13 March 2002.
189 E. Emerson, 'What is Normalisation?', in *Normalisation: A Reader for the Nineties*, (eds) H. Smith and H. Brown (London: Tavistock/Routledge, 1992), p. 14.
190 L. Ward, "Forward", in *Normalisation: A Reader for the Nineties*, (eds) H. Brown and H. Smith. (London: Tavistock/Routledge, 1992), p. 4.
191 D. Towell, 'An ordinary life: comprehensive locally-based residential services for mentally handicapped', project paper no. 24, reprint (London: King's Fund, 1982).
192 K. Stalker, *'Share the Care': An Evaluation of Family Based Respite Care Services* (London: Jessica Kingsley, 1990), p. 23.

3   Barriers to communication

COMMUNICATING WITH SERVICE USERS

The tradition of social work is one of giving advice, carrying out assessments, report writing, and advocacy to promote choice and independence. Communication is therefore at the very core of social work activities. In more recent years, the language of community care has called for professionals to develop a greater range of communication skills and interpersonal abilities to help aid users. Makaton, a simple system of signed communication, has been developed to aid communication with non-verbal people. However, it remains the case that despite much emphasis placed on communication during the training of social workers, in practice professionals are often limited in their abilities, through a lack of practical experience. Classroom teaching emphasises how social workers *ought* to communicate, what they should *know* and be striving to achieve, but much of the evidence suggests this is not the reality of field practice.[193] Such limitations on the part of the professional raise serious questions such as:

- How do social workers communicate with service users?
- Do professionals attempt to adjust their approach to communication when dealing with different user groups?
- What communication skills are effective in what setting and why?[194]

Some answers to these problems can be found in social psychology and behavioural theory, which offer aids for dealing with verbal, non-verbal and symbolic communication.

INTERPERSONAL COMMUNICATION: SYMBOLIC, NON-VERBAL AND VERBAL

Having a dialogue that involves expressive and receptive communication is a two-way process, which means that certain stages in the development of communication have followed distinct milestones of speech and language acquisition. Normally, for example, children interact with others from birth. In the early months this development ranges from vocalisations allowing an understanding about how the child is feeling (crying demonstrates distress or pain) and from around 6 months onwards gestures and signs are developed. The final stage is when the child produces actual linguistic forms to convey his or her intentions and feelings and by this time the child realises that communicative ability can evoke responses from adults.[195] Table 3 summarises this process of speech development.

The goal of spoken language development is to equip a child with the most adaptable, generalised and acceptable communication skills possible. Children with mild to moderate learning disabilities go through these stages but at a much slower rate. Some may be delayed in their language development due either to cognitive impairment or to an unrewarding language environment. In many cases problems with the early stages of communication development can be an indication that the child has problems in other areas of its mental development.

The role that a parent of a child with learning disabilities has in this process is critical to the way in which the child progresses. A considerable literature is beginning to appear discussing the important role parents play in language acquisition and communication development of children with learning disabilities. Mitchell (1987) observes that parent–infant interaction for the most part is a process that should be led by the infant.[196] Burford (1988) advocates in favour of this approach where there is a parent–child interaction with a profoundly disabled child, and goes on to extend his

Table 3 Milestones of speech and language acquisition (at average age)

Birth	*Vocalisations*
6 months	Babble
10 months	Reduplications appear: 'ma-ma', 'da-da'
1 year	One-word sentences
18 months	Two-word utterances
20 months	Telegrammatic speech
2 years	Pre-sleep monologues
2.5 years	50-word lexicon, 5-word sentences, use of personal pronoun
3 years	Plurals established, 250 words
3.5 years	'p', 'b', 'm', 'w', 'h' pronounced; how and why questions
4 years	Tells story; still morphological errors
4.5 years	't', 'k', 'd', 'ng', 'y' pronounced; asks what words mean
5.5 years	'f', 'z', 's', 'v' pronounced
6.5 years	'sh', 'zh', 'I', 'th' pronounced; adult morphology complete
	Listens to another's standpoint in conversation
8 years	'ch', 'r', 'wh' pronounced

Source: B. Fraser, 'Communicating with People with Learning Disabilities', in *Seminars in the Psychiatry of Learning Disabilities*, ed. Oliver Russell (London: Gaskell and the Royal College of Psychiatrists, 1997), p. 180

theory to include severely disabled adults. Burford's 'Communication through Movement' approach proposes that:

> The basic principles are to try to find out some history of the person with a profound handicap (for example, what his preferred way of signalling is; what he finds enjoyable from adults), and then to watch and spot 'what's on offer' (that includes assuming intentionality; unless proved otherwise, every movement and every silence means something); and to be particularly sensitive to the pace or rhythm of interaction.[197]

Kiernan and Reid (1987) offer a method for assessing children with learning disabilities, and calculate their ability to communicate through the *Preverbal Communication Schedule* (PVCS).[198] Kiernan and Reid developed this procedure by assessing a child's interests and preferences through

- expressions of emotion using non-verbal communication;
- interaction: the extent to which the child socially and emotionally interacts;
- the ability to respond to stimuli such as singing to music and infant–parent communication.

Fraser (1997) argues that:

> The overall message . . . is that even those who are most profoundly disabled do produce communicative acts, and that parents and care staff can be very skilled in reacting to often very opaque communications. The professional ought to be at least as skilled.[199]

He suggests professionals should be informed about a variety of techniques that can be used in order to overcome communication barriers when dealing with individuals who have profound learning disabilities. His suggestions are summarised in Figure 2.

The present study revealed that the responses given by professionals when asked about communicating with non-verbal individuals did not differ significantly whether they were social workers or had been clinically trained. Clare is a clinical psychologist specialising in communicating with people with learning disabilities. She has worked in the department for the past seven years. Her approach typifies that of many professionals, both within the health and the social care sections:

> 'I try to find ways of communicating that are as clear as possible for non-verbal people. We start from a disadvantage point which is to do with the power imbalance inherent between us and the user. Naturally this creates difficulties between both parties. Users may ask a question

Figure 2 Communication with people with a profound learning disability

Make it enjoyable – practise where the person produces most (e.g. outings).
Do it regularly.
Do not cramp your style by too much formality.
Be an opportunist – sing, act, whistle, change your voice, gear and speech.
Use consistent labels.
Take small steps, and do not reach for a level far beyond the person's development.
Remember to signal vigorously with your face and do not forget that the person may not signal back.
If the person is not looking, he or she is not listening.
Give him time to answer.
Cue her by her name.
The onus is on you to ensure you are understood.
The behaviour of the person with a learning disability is the starting point.
Relate to the person's disability rather than his or her chronological age. (Note: this does not fit the normalisation philosophy of Wolfensberger.)
Always assume intentionality – that the behaviour, however strange, means something.

Source: B. Fraser, 'Communicating with People with a Profound Learning Disability', in *Seminars in the Psychiatry of Learning Disabilities*, ed. Oliver Russell (London: Gaskell and the Royal College of Psychiatrists, 1997), p. 184.

that has a depth of meaning for them, but which we do not fully understand. We have to find new ways to help them in such circumstances. Empower them to develop skills that will give them more ways to make their choices known. What we can offer is shaped by the organisation as the provider agency. The organisation chooses what it offers.

Communicating with people with learning disabilities falls into two areas, the macro and the micro. On the micro, individual level, I embark upon a period of discussion with the person looking at what they think will benefit them. It sounds good but the reality with non-verbal users is of course very difficult in lots of ways. These themes we are talking about today, choice and inclusion, are subjective and abstract concepts, which the average person in the street has problems grasping let alone someone with learning disabilities. What I try to bring to my work is imagination and creativity. Part of the problem is trying to elicit a response from the user that says *I understand you*. I feel it is very important to repeat that rationale behind what you are doing and invite people's comments as much as they can comment.

Having other people involved is important. It offers other perspectives in the sense that they are different perspectives from those of the staff. That's where partnership working, having health and social care professionals working together in the one building, has been such a success for us in this borough, we're very lucky in that respect. Parents, carers and advocates can all make valuable contributions as well. On a personal level I'm interested to hear what people have to say. For one it broadens the process and deepens my understanding of the person I am attempting to help. It is always unhelpful when staff members believe they have the sole answer, usually based on very little evidence beyond it's what they think is right for that individual. This can be a process of degeneration rather than having a positive collaborative approach. There is one difficulty and it is an experience I have had on a number of occasions, it's when the user doesn't want anyone else involved, that can be very difficult. When this happens it means the negotiation begins again.'

The difficulty with what Clare is saying is that she fails to grapple effectively with the problem of communication, and instead skates over the difficulties choosing to talk in general terms.

With the emphasis on moving those people with learning disabilities in institutional care to community settings, such as smaller group homes, comes the need for methods to tackle many problems associated with the attempt to generate a sense of community. Communication skills are crucial to the success of living in small group homes in the community, and without frameworks in place which actively support people with learning disabilities they can fail in their attempts to become part of the wider community. Those most likely to want to live independently are individuals with mild to moderate learning disabilities, but who are none the less deficient in a variety of cognitive and communication abilities. Language is a complex process requiring skills of articulation and comprehension. People with learning disabilities commonly experience an inability to organise the structures that are needed to communicate clearly. They quite often lack the capacity to design information and present it adequately in an extended discourse. Dennis, the father of an autistic son, to some extent blames the lack of educational opportunity for people with learning disabilities to develop greater communication skills. He spoke about the difficulties his son experiences:

'We need to remember my son was born at a time when people with learning difficulties were pigeon-holed. Not a great deal of effort was given over to those who couldn't communicate. In those days he was classed as severe educationally subnormal. Then in 1972 the responsibility changed from health to education. They said he was incapable of being educated. His ability though is high in some ways but then his social skills and relating to people isn't that good. He often has inappropriate behaviour – he's autistic. Communication is a real problem for us and so the depth of his knowledge and understanding is difficult to assess. He can't read but he can identify words, we think it's to do with the patterns and shapes. He has a difficult speech pattern to understand. He uses speech and Makaton. He automatically signs when he speaks but his ability to sign isn't great. His needs outweigh his ability to communicate them. It's difficult, it isn't an easy one to find a solution to. His behaviour, well like most people with autism, routine is very important to him and he finds dealing with the unexpected very difficult. It is a real problem if a service lets him down, transport for example, his anxiety goes up and it can take as long as a month for him to recover. I think a real part of his frustration is the fact he can't communicate his feelings.'

Fraser (1997) suggests:

> ... communicative exchange is more than a series of unrelated speaking turns, there is a logical progression and a competent listener keeps track of the topic to make an appropriate contribution. It is important to establish reference: the listener must determine what an expression refers to and the speaker must ensure that the reference identification is possible. There must be an appropriate use of ties, i.e. linguistic devices such as 'this' or 'that', which make sentences coherent.[200]

Fraser argues that utterances give signals which can be understood; if they are not he offers the methods of *reflection* and *correction*. Reflection, he suggests, is not a strength of people with learning disabilities, and trying to get their point across in conversation can often result in their becoming distressed and anxious. Although unable to reflect on the causes of the conversational incompetence, the individual may be aware there is something 'wrong' with his or her conversation such as inappropriate language or disjointed ideas. When the person takes steps to rectify the situation it may result in their becoming flustered, feeling out of their depth, or the meaning of what they are trying to say may be lost completely. This in turn has the potential of triggering disturbed and challenging behaviour.[201]

Symbolic communication

A significant amount of social work literature has appeared emphasising the importance of symbolic communication, highlighting the significance attached to behaviour, actions and communication. Symbolic communication is a process whereby potential meanings are attached to the surrounding environment. A warm smile from a receptionist and offer of a seat convey respect and concern and is a symbolic interaction, giving a sense of being both welcomed and wanted. In contrast, being ignored while the receptionist deals with numerous telephone calls or other people, displays a lack of respect and can cause feelings of intrusion, being a nuisance or in the way.[202] D'Ardenne and Mahtani (1989) observe that the symbolic aspects of the physical environment can often prove a powerful statement of what they term the professional's *transcultural viewpoint*.[203] That is to say, the physical environment can convey other messages such as race and class. Pictures showing different ethnic groups, for example, are more welcoming to clients of differing ethnic origins and demonstrate another aspect of non-verbal symbolic communication.

Non-verbal communication

Non-verbal communication is as powerful in the meanings it can carry as symbolic communication. Sign language, body movement, facial expression and gaze are some of the main characteristics that go to make up non-verbal communication. There is a substantial literature about non-verbal body language that tells us that while verbal communication is concerned with directly conveying information, non-verbal communication is about feelings and attitude. A problem that non-verbal communication has is the difficulty it can present when trying to understand and interpret the situation, due to inherent ambiguity. Interactions between professionals and users are sometimes fraught with difficulty because of such ambiguous non-verbal interaction between them. For the majority of professionals who participated in this study, non-verbal interaction was an insurmountable barrier; for example, one social worker said:

> 'The feeling of controlling the whole thing is a profoundly difficult one. The best way to involve non-verbal severely disabled people is on a one to one, but we need to acknowledge that some communication problems just can't be overcome.'

Lishman (1994) offers a method for overcoming these obstacles, where professionals adopt a mode of non-verbal behaviour that fits with the particular situation they are involved with at the time. For example:

> Children seem particularly aware of and sensitive to non-verbal behaviour. In working with deaf people our posture, position and facial expressions will be particularly important; with blind people our voice, tone and touch. In residential work non-verbal behaviour is constantly on view.[204]

Non-verbal communication is divided into two categories:

(1) *Proxemics*: which is concerned with the distance people like between them;
(2) *Kinesics*: which is to do with expression, movement, eye contact and gesture.

Distance, closeness, proximity, posture and touch are all-important aspects to consider in any discourse on non-verbal communication. An example of *proxemics* would be giving a hug or pat conveying understanding and support to the user. In a similar way, *kinesics* deals with eye contact and facial expressions, and has several important functions during conversation. It is known that in conversation one participant looks at the other more when he or she is listening than when speaking. A participant looks at the other when she or he finishes speaking and looks away at the beginning of speaking, signalling the beginning and end of the conversation.[205] Facial expressions can give non-verbal clues; frowning can be interpreted as criticism, a bored expression communicates distance. Facial expression is directly linked to responsiveness and is a two-way process. Interestingly, smiling is an expression that is cross-cultural: across all cultures smiling conveys a non-threatening approach that is both positive and friendly.[206] Eye contact, body language and facial expressions tell a lot about how the individual is feeling. A glazed expression, a fixed smile, looking around the room or frequent shifts in position, can convey discomfort with the relationship. The reason for this may be that communication is not being understood on the part of the user or the purpose of the interaction is not clear.

The *principles* of communicating with individuals who have mild learning disabilities apply equally to those with profound learning disabilities. It is important to have some knowledge about the person and her or his likes and dislikes, and this helps to make communication more interesting and stimulating. Communication with people with severe disabilities means looking for what the person has to offer in the form of communication and waiting for clues. Undoubtedly, as with any individual, the closer and longer-lasting the relationship the greater the probability of understanding their needs and preferences. Consider 'Personal reflections on voice', the account of one mother's personal experience of her relationship with her young severely disabled, non-verbal son – Kim.

Personal reflections on voice[207]

'I started to think about the different ways in which we communicate with each other some eight years ago when my son Kim lost the ability to communicate in a manner which was language-based.

Watching Kim day in, day out, I slowly became aware that his loss of a language-based means of communication did not make a fundamental difference to our relationship. I realised that I was easily able to interpret his needs, his desires, his preferences through his body language. Did his eyes look tense? Did he feel tense? What did his eyes look like? Was he alert and interested? Was he lethargic and disinterested? If he appeared to be low in energy was that connected to tiring seizures or was he demonstrating a lack of interest and/or dislike with regards to what was going on around him? I began to see that communication between us was not exclusive to him and me as mother and son. Many other people who enjoyed his company and spent regular time with him had access to exactly the same kind of relationship. I also realised that such communication was a part of all relationships but because we were so focused on language-based communication we paid little attention.

As the years went by and Kim became weaker and more frequently "poorly" his overt communication became increasingly more subtle. In spite of this it never became less definite, the signs of what he required and/or preferred were there up to, and including, his death. It seemed that there was a continuum of communication, dependent only on the drawing of breath . . . As he withdrew into himself more, I followed his lead and spoke less to him. The communication between us did not lessen, it simply adapted to meet the changing needs of the situation. It seemed a high level of communication was possible without language. Language only became necessary to convey his wishes to others, to ensure that he was getting what he wanted in any situation involving the "outside world".

Due to the subtle way in which Kim expressed himself it was very easy for others to ignore his preferences and to justify this by claiming that either they could not understand him, or he had little understanding, or he did not communicate. Whilst it is impossible to say how much and in what way he did understand language this did not necessarily provide a block to listening to him. To understand Kim took some time and a willingness to do so in addition to a degree of openness to possibilities different from the norm. With these factors in place understanding was guaranteed.

It is difficult to find words to talk about, to explore through language, a means of communication which is not language-based. It is easy to dismiss such an exploration, to have it put down as the imaginings of a fond parent.'

The experiences and feelings of parents interviewed during this study often mirrored the words of Kim's mother. What was significant, and can be seen from the following discussion, is that for some parents there was a difficulty in determining what the barriers to communication actually were. Because the discussion was about their sons and daughters the responses were highly subjective, for example, "I know my child and what he wants." Margaret, the mother of a profoundly disabled man who has autism, said:

'In some ways when things are very obvious he can be clear about indicating his wishes, he's always clear when he wants something to drink, or some food. He pushes your hand towards what he wants, it's that simple. If he wants to go out he will make very definite moves. He doesn't use any kind of speech, but that doesn't stop him when he wants to do something like last weekend we went for a walk, believe me he was quite definite about going uphill when mom wanted to go downhill. He led me on a nice walk around the park. One of his strengths is that he knows where he is; often rather than being at his residential home he will turn up on my doorstep.

When he can't make himself understood that's when his behaviour becomes challenging. When he gets distressed he will start biting his wrist or hand, this happens when he gets confused or unhappy in part. We never know what has triggered it; perhaps it is something that has happened a long time ago, we just don't know. Despite this I would say he does have a lot of autonomy, I have to allow him his space. Relationships are quite important to him but he can also completely ignore people. I've never been able to figure that one out.'

Other parents also described their sons' and daughters' ability to make themselves understood through their non-verbal interaction. With the example of Peter a father tells how he felt it was not communication difficulties that held his son back:

'I don't talk about it as a communication problem, that's such a defeatist attitude to adopt, at least for me it is. He does communicate but just not with speech and I would prefer to talk about it as a combination of three things, negotiation, free will and coercion. My son Peter already attends college and as many classes as he can. He can't speak very well and his ideas are often very disjointed. The staff are very good at the college, and they also listen to what Peter is trying to say through his body language and his movements. They always try to include his choices in class but sadly sometimes certainly with this council it is about money not communication that stops him developing.'

Verbal communication

Verbal communication is oral or spoken communication and is often thought of in the sense of asking questions and getting answers, which poses a problem for professionals who often seek to avoid question-and-answer sessions for fear of putting answers into the mouths of service users. It has been suggested that careful thought should be given to the approach taken. Some of the key questions which may arise include:

- How can the information be gained in a neutral way?
- Could the question be shorter or paraphrased?
- Is there an alternative method that could be used instead of asking a question?
- What may happen in the question–answer interaction?
- Is a relationship based on power where the professional is perceived as knowing what is best for the user?[208]

Winston is a care manager in the learning disability team who spoke about his experiences, and the importance of having a clear framework in which to operate a question-and-answer session:

'. . . other ways are a mixture of groups, face-to-face interviews and also questionnaires. This means involving other groups from the voluntary sector and advocates. An important problem to be aware of is the framework of the questions to get good feedback. I would say it is up to people at a local level as to how far they take it. In the past day centres have worked with users to get responses to questions. But they also included observed behaviour by the staff in the centre who knew the users well, and felt they could interpret the users' behaviour. They knew them over time. If the user has had limited experiences of services and being involved then they will have limited expectations, but if they don't have limited experiences their choices and expectations would be bigger like getting a job. The majority were happy with what they were getting, it's pretty good. The day centres are good, they work towards getting the most out of the users.'

Focusing, summarising, confrontation and having an awareness of barriers to communication can all help. Focusing involves concentrating on what the individual is saying in order to see potentially conflicting ideas. People with learning disabilities often present professionals with wide-ranging themes during the course of a discussion. Focusing picks up and separates out the themes, and provides a way of getting to grips with a greater emotional depth, enabling the worker to see the *core messages* coming from the person. Focusing allows the professional to ask the question: *What is the user really concerned about and how can I help him or her?* It is often true that what the client is worried about is not what is raised in an interview. Egan (1986)[209] believes that summarising can aid focusing in the sense that it clarifies what the user has said, selecting the key issues and conveying the essence of the discussion. Summarising allows the professional to check that she or he understands the content and feeling of what the user has been saying. Egan suggests that summarising helps the individual to clarify his or her own perspective and enables her or him to develop alternatives. Confrontation is defined as having a hostile attitude, and has connotations of aggression, destructiveness and personal attack.[210] However, Carkhuff (1969)[211] believes that confronting the service users is useful, because it helps them to understand discrepancies in their own behaviour, feelings or thinking.

Susan is a service user who offered an example of how confrontation, if it had been used by her social worker, would have helped Susan understand what she wanted to do, instead of always agreeing with what the social worker said. Susan explained:

> 'My social worker, yes she does help me with college and stuff like that. She helps me with transport and she helped get me to college yeah. I don't know about college yet, I start next week yeah. She tells me I'll make lots of friends and I'm doing cooking, reading and learning how to write properly. Learn how to stand up for yourself and say no, that's what she said. I've got this problem, I say yes to everything. It's got me into trouble. I say yes when I talk to my social worker all the time about things and then go home and tell my mom I don't want to do it. Like at college I'd say yes and then go home and get into trouble from mom and college rings me up and I get in trouble and all. I don't really like college that much anyway.'

There are a number of conditions that are believed to have the potential for blocking communication such as the physical environment: having a television on during a home visit, or being in a hot stuffy room, for example. Interruptions distract and disrupt the flow of conversation and it should be remembered that there are limits to the amount of verbal information a person can take in. It is essential to be clear about what is being said and what is being understood: unchecked assumptions lead to misunderstandings. Similarly there is the danger of categorising people on the grounds of nationality, race, class, occupation, age and appearance. Finally, where there is no common language an interpreter will be needed, but having a third party can also produce further problems including inaccuracies, translation bias and distortion.[212]

Individuals with profound communication problems are those most likely to be restricted in their opportunities and access to services of their choosing. As the previous discussion indicates, one reason for this is the time it takes to work with people with profound disabilities to enable them to communicate their choices. Communication is both *expressive* and *receptive,* a two-way process where some people may express but cannot receive or understand what is being communicated to them. The organisation Choices at Makfield is a group that supports people with profound learning difficulties to express their wishes. It offers the following example, which it says shows that, with time and persistence, this question may be successfully addressed:

> *Anna [a support worker] describes how Richard has made choices:*
>
> 'Richard is a young man who is quite mobile, and has severe learning difficulties. He has had regular sessions from his home. Staff meet for breakfast at his house. Knowing that he enjoys music they make regular use of the local music library. Richard now smiles and makes eye contact with his support workers. He is beginning to assert himself. By rocking in his wheelchair, he indicated that he wishes to walk home from the shops.'[213]

In Liverpool at the Step Out Project, which supports people with learning disabilities into work experience, there is a profoundly disabled man called Brian who overcame his communication difficulties so that staff were able to understand the kind of work he wanted to do:

> [having] been in his work placement for six months . . . Brian indicated by reaching out to touch the photocopier and imitating its noise that he would also like to develop his skills in that area.[214]

It would seem that given these examples people with profound difficulties can be empowered to make valid choices, even with limited communication. However, they fail to inform us about how the observers arrive at their conclusions. Rather they offer a positive yet flyaway explanation with no real evidence to support them. Individuals who cannot express themselves well through verbal communication run the risk of *learned helplessness* resulting in a belief that nothing they do or say will make a difference even in the routine of daily life.[215]

A report produced by the Foundation for People with Learning Disabilities, *Everyday Lives, Everyday Choices*, believes that the challenge is having a shared understanding of what the individual wants to communicate, arguing that:

> challenging behaviour is still too often seen as a problem which must be managed, rather than as a communicative act needing to be interpreted and understood.[216]

The report continues by offering the example of a person who was taken to the pub for a social outing, but who repeatedly ran to the pub door and growled. Staff coaxed him back encouraging him to remain, but what the individual was really attempting to communicate was his displeasure with the environment. Perhaps it was too smoky, or too loud, and he wanted to go home. The illustration demonstrates the need to listen and observe acts such as scratching, grunting noises, taps and even silence. These are ways non-verbal people communicate which staff should seek to interpret. The direction of the eyes, facial and bodily expressions, all are clues by which people express themselves. This all takes time which professionals say they cannot afford. If inclusion and choice are to become realities in the lives of people with high support needs then real challenges lie ahead.

Many keyworkers and residential home managers spoke about their frustration at not being able to find enough time during their normal working day to experiment with different ways of communicating with their users. Errol, a residential home manager with many years' experience of learning disabilities, sees the problem not only in terms of time, but also as a lack of creativity among professionals together with a lack of willingness to commit resources:

> 'We have a limited amount of time during our day to spend with our users, and it's not only about the length of time you spend with your client, it's about how creative you can be to communicate with that person. I have had many ideas I have put to the senior managers in the department about this, and how we could experiment with different methods of communicating choices by our users. There are many examples of how to approach helping an individual with multiple disabilities to make choices, such as arranging for a user to communicate by means of blowing on an especially adapted switch. Another way is using infrared pads that go under the person's arms. We could then show images on a screen and they could squeeze the pad to indicate their choice. This can even be developed for users who can only lie on the floor because their disability is so profound. More capable users, but still without speech, can touch colours on a screen to indicate their choice; symbols such as the car symbol to let their keyworker know they want to go out in the car today. You see, communicating with people with severe communication disabilities is all about creativity. Sadly this council have said they can't support this form of technology because of the cost.'

COMMUNICATION AND EQUIPMENT

Valuing People is one of the first government papers to acknowledge that a main obstacle to the successful participation of people with learning disabilities in service planning has been, and continues to be, communication. It expects professionals and organisations working with individuals to create policies that will achieve greater advancement of communication, and one suggestion made is through more extensive use of new technology. They argue that such technology can more readily assist people to express choices in a clearer and more accessible manner.

Roberta is a speech and language therapist working for the department. She spoke about her experience around communication and the importance equipment played. Roberta said:

'Asking people to become involved in planning their own services when they have communication problems, it's a difficult one. We try a variety of ways to help people understand, including symbols and Makaton to get the message and the importance of what is happening over. We also have contracts. These contracts are talked about in terms of non-verbal and pre-verbal contracts, their function is to look at the aims of what we have set out to do. So, for example, we may be attempting to include someone to make a decision when there is need to change his or her service. There may be some clinical reason why the service must change and we want them to be a part of that change process. In terms of involving users in the decision-making about planning we haven't done very much in this council. It is a difficult bulk of work with pre- and non-verbal people; we try various routes such as involving their keyworker. That way we all have a shared sense of responsibility. I would say most recent consultation amounts to lip-service. It's my experience that in the speech and language therapy centre, we are seen simply as a translation service. People who write complicated documents must understand we are not translators for their work. They must use simple plain English to get their message across.

We have users with learning disabilities that we link up with who don't have speech but do understand speech. This can be due to one form of neurological damage or another. We have systems and terms of reference that we work to. Let me give you an example of this work. Dinner for instance, we use a spoon: a spoon is an easy way for the non-verbal people to identify with so as to communicate the fact they are hungry. The day centre is doing a lot of work like this, but it's very slow and takes a great deal of time. We are constantly exploring new ways to help our users communicate. Only one user in the council has an electronic communicator aid, which allows speech by touching a keyboard, you know like Stephen Hawking has. This has increased communication beyond our expectations. It proved to us what we have known all along about the level of his intelligence. These machines are very expensive and that's a real problem. We raise the users' expectations and then we can't come through for them because of budget restrictions. Our user only got the electronic aid because he had a lucky break. Budgets impact directly on choice and services. Politicians and policy makers are aware of the value these aids can bring, but how many times do you hear about them telling us about cutbacks, how can social service departments pay for them? I can think of at least four service users I see who could desperately do with one of these aids.

The budgets in this department are still as they were before we had partnership working pretty separate. There was talk about pooled funding but I guess that's in the future. It is understandable then when parents are seen as a problem, especially when they demand expensive equipment like this. We try our best to tell them about the problems to do with financing and in a way they can understand, but it's very difficult especially when they are often so angry with you. I can really understand it and you do feel for them. If I had a child who I thought could benefit from having one of these communication aids, I think I'd be shouting as well. There needs to be a genuine dialogue not the polarisation we have at the moment. It's difficult with the financial constraints we are all working under in the learning disabilities section.'

The government states in *Valuing People* that it is committed to spend extra funding for new initiatives such as equipment to aid communication, and asks both social services and the NHS to

Improve and expand community equipment services. By 2004 the Government expects health and social services to integrate their community equipment services, and increase by 50% the number of people benefiting from them.[217]

But there are communication difficulties that are specific to some people with learning disabilities that have implications, not only for the professionals working in the area, but also for researchers.

GOVERNMENT POLICY AND COMMUNICATION: THE EVIDENCE REVEALED

Political rhetoric at a central and local level has emphasised the importance of the consultation process by social service departments. However, progress to develop ways of involving service users in planning services has been slow, and it remains unclear how best to consult users, especially those with profound learning disabilities.[218] The difficulty has been underlined by recent studies that have shown:

• 50% of the total population of people with learning disabilities living in Britain today have communication difficulties according to the definitions used and the sample surveyed.[219]

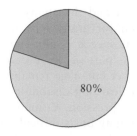
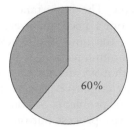

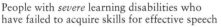

People with *severe* learning disabilities who have failed to acquire skills for effective speech

People with *mild* disabilities who have some skills in symbolic communication

Source: Foundation for People with Learning Disabilities, *Learning Disabilities: the Fundamental Facts*, researched and written by Eric Emerson, Chris Hatton, David Felce and Glynis Murphy (FPLD, 2001).

Figure 3 Communication in people with learning disabilities

- About 80% of people with severe learning disabilities fail to acquire effective speech.[220]
- Some 60% of people with learning disabilities overall have some skills in symbolic communication, such as speech, signs or picture symbols.[221]
- Around 20% have no verbal communication skills but do demonstrate intentional communication.[222]
- Clear evidence can be established of a person's intention to communicate and an expectation of a response.[223]
- About 20% have no intentional communication skills.[224]

In other words, the government has a policy of communication and involvement, but at least 20% of people with learning disabilities are known not to have a means of communication interaction.

COMMUNICATION AND THE PROBLEMS OF RESEARCHING THE VIEWS OF PEOPLE WITH LEARNING DISABILITIES

Consulting any group of users about the services they receive is daunting enough, but consulting people with learning disabilities has the added dilemmas of communication and cognitive understanding. Among the common drawbacks for users trying to communicate their ideas about choice, and the type of services they want, is a lack of experience at being asked their opinion. Social as well as communication skills may be underdeveloped, and they may experience difficulty getting views across. The ability to express and communicate choice is of overriding importance to the whole process of consultation, service planning and social inclusion. The importance of communication and the ability to communicate one's needs in everyday life is taken for granted by most of us most of the time. While acknowledging that speech is just one aspect of daily communication, it is such a significant part of our everyday experience that we do not even think about it, yet language remains a highly complex cognitive process. For people with learning disabilities there are the extra problems of comprehension and expression. Communication is a two-way process but one where *reception* may be as difficult as *expression*. If an advocate is included, having another person involved in the process is in itself filled with potential challenges. It is not only understanding what is said that is the problem, but also the hinterland that lies behind it.

In the case of the present study, there was a commitment to provide full and accessible information about this study to potential participants so that they had a clear understanding about the intended aims, outcomes, how the interviews would be carried out, the terms under which people were to be involved, and the subjects of interest that would be discussed with them. This provided clear information that enabled participants to make an informed decision about whether they wished to be included. For anyone engaging in research in this area, there are formidable communication problems to be overcome if people representing the full spectrum of ability are to be included. However, even before interpersonal communication is attempted, institutional pressures may seriously reduce the prospect of success and jeopardise the most serious attempts to prepare the ground well for users to make choices on the basis of information.

NOTES

193 W. Schwartz, 'Thoughts from Abroad: Some Perspectives on the Practice of Social Work', *Social Work Today* (1973) 14.

194 J. Lishman, *Communication in Social Work* (Basingstoke/London: Macmillan, 1994) p. 3.

195 B. Fraser, 'Communicating with People with Learning Disabilities', in *Seminars in the Psychiatry of Learning Disabilities*, (ed.) Oliver Russell (London: Gaskell/the Royal College of Psychiatrists, 1997), p. 180.

196 D. R. Mitchell, 'Parents' Interactions for Mentally Handicapped People', in *Mentally Handicapped People,* (eds) M. Beveridge, G. Conti-Ramsden and I. Leudar (London: Chapman and Hall: 1987) pp. 274–99.

197 B. Burford, 'Action cycles: rhythmic actions for engagement with children and young adults with profound mental handicap', *European Journal of Special Needs Education*, 3, pp. 189–206.

198 C. Kiernan and B. Reid, *The Preverbal Communication Schedule (PVCS)* (Windsor: NFER/Nelson 1987).

199 Fraser, 'Communicating with People', p. 188.

200 ibid., p. 185.

201 ibid., p. 186.

202 Lishman, *Communication*, p. 15.
203 P. D'Ardenne and A. Mahtani, *Transcultural Counselling in Action* (London: Sage, 1989), p. 53.
204 Lishman, *Communication*, p. 20.
205 A. Kendon, 'Some Functions of Gaze-Direction in Social Interaction', in M. Argyle (ed.), *Social Encounters: Readings in Social Interaction* (Harmondsworth: Penguin, 1973, repr 1976).
206 M. Argyle, *Social Encounters: Readings in Social Interaction* (Harmondsworth: Penguin, 1978).
207 Pippa Murray, 'Personal Reflections on Voice', in *Telling Our Own Stories: Reflections on Family Life in a Disabling World*, (eds) Pippa Murray and Jill Penman (Sheffield: Parents with Attitude, 2000), pp. 251–4.
208 Lishman, *Communication*, p. 24.
209 G. Egan, *The Skilled Helper: A Systematic Approach to Effective Helping* (Monterey, CA: Brookes/Cole, 1986) p. 173.
210 *Chambers English Dictionary* (1988).
211 R. R. Carkhuff, *Helping and Human Relations* (New York: Holt, 1969), p. 73.
212 Lishman, *Communication*, pp. 31–3.
213 The Mental Health Foundation, 'Working with People with Severe, Profound and Multiple Learning Difficulties', Bulletin 5 (London: MHF, 1999), p. 3.
214 ibid., p. 4.
215 M. E. P. Seligman, *Helplessness on Depressions, Development, and Death* (San Francisco: Freeman, 1975).
216 "*Let them Speak*": www.communitycare.co.uk
217 ibid., p. 52.
218 S. McIver, *Obtaining the Views of Users of Health Services* (London: King's Fund, 1992). D. Sperlinger and L. McAuslane, 'Listening to Users of Services for People with Dementia', *Clinical Psychology Forum* (1994) 72: 2–4. J. Jenkins, and L. Grey, 'Multidisciplinary Audit by a Service for People with Learning Disabilities: Quality Assurance and Customers' Views', *Clinical Psychology Forum* (1994) 69: 22–9.
219 A. Van der Gaag, 'Communication Skills and Adults with Learning Disabilities: Eliminating Professional Myopia', *British Journal of Learning Disabilities* (1998) 26: 88–93.
220 E. E. Garcia and E. D. De Haven, 'Use of Operant Techniques in the Establishment of and Generalization of Language: a Review and Analysis', *American Journal of Mental Deficiency* (1974) 79: 169–78.
221 McLean, Brady and McLean, 'Reported Communication Abilities'.
222 T. Iacono, M. Carter, and J. Hook, 'Identification of Intentional Communication in Students with Severe and Multiple Disabilities', *Augmentative and Alternative Communication* (1998) 14: 102–14.
223 McLean, Brady and McLean, 'Reported Communication Abilities'.
224 ibid.

4 Strategies for implementing normalisation and citizenship

TOWARDS A NEW CULTURE OF SOCIAL CARE

Much research literature in recent years owes its origins to the considerable confusion surrounding the process of turning the ideological concept of *community care,* steeped as it is in political rhetoric, into a workable social policy, especially in the context of resource constraints. The main concern for social services professionals has been and remains under-funding and over-spending. Examples of under-funding and over-spending are best seen with residential units which house high-needs and high-dependency service users. Relocating users who are moved from larger units, especially the old-style long-stay hospitals, and housing them in smaller group homes accommodating two or three people, presents challenges for even the most creative budget controller. Service planners and commissioners are keen to find alternative methods for delivering the same services as economically and cost-effectively as possible.

During the early 1990s, the way in which social services were delivered dramatically changed. While the state remained the sole financier for social care provision, it sought to reduce its role as the lead provider.[225] One of the most interesting aspects of this shift was the unpredictability that went with it. No one, for example, could have imagined in 1990, the change in the nature of the GP to that of fund holder or the introduction of a contract culture. Contracting for human services had been a part of social policy in the United States for more than 20 years, and in Britain was introduced as part of the NHS & Community Care Act (1990). Roles underwent fundamental changes as a result of the new policy and the idea behind the introduction of contracts was to formalise arrangements that had hitherto been created on an informal basis.[226] The policy of contracting for social care was only part of a greater shift in the delivery of public services, such as the adoption of market principles from the private sector. The Conservative government was keen to roll back the state as the main provider of social welfare, and promote the private and voluntary sectors as key providers, with the idea of reducing government expenditure.[227] The government believed that the market-place was the superior and most efficient arena for delivering more choice and higher-quality services. It justified its approach by suggesting that providers were essentially self-interested, thus making it impossible for professional ethics to regulate systems of public provision. At the same time the core objective of the new community care policy was to check the haemorrhage of public funds which had developed in the wake of the changes in social security regulations in 1983 intended to stimulate the private market in residential care.[228] In this sense, community care was positioned somewhere between concerns about the social security budget and pressures on the NHS, and the reforms were not solely, or even principally, about the development of care in the community *per se*.[229]

The move towards market principles formed part of a wider movement with similar developments happening in other European countries.[230] However, Britain was unique in this venture, because it was the only country to try out so many aspects of market principles across the broad spectrum of public service provision.

The introduction of the legislation in 1990 set out three aspects for its vision:

(1) the establishment of a purchaser/provider split;
(2) an increase in the amount of independent provision;
(3) the regulation of providers by the use of contracts.[231]

The Conservative government believed that separating purchasing from providing was necessary to ensure that the respective interests of users and providers were separately represented.[232] It suggested that being in a position to offer a larger supply of services would lead to more flexibility and responsiveness to the needs of those individuals and groups using the services. At the same time this would help to create more efficiency via contracts. Establishing contracts imposed stringent checks on quality and a more vigorous approach to management. The idea behind the development of the *enabling authority* was linked to a more precise tailoring of services to needs and was not solely about contracting out, privatisation or even cost-effectiveness. The government wanted local authorities to move away from institutional and residential care and towards domiciliary care; however, the majority of public and independent provision was largely residential and nursing care. In the United States, where there was a much longer tradition of social services marketisation, the results of studies had shown that contracting for human services, with specialist providers, often resulted in the organisations becoming monopolistic, which ironically was the opposite effect to the one intended by the British government. It also meant the choice of supplier was more often than not limited.[233]

There were other competing demands on social service departments such as the information and monitoring requirements of the Social Services Inspectorate, the regional health authorities, and the Department of Health as well as the Audit Commission. Most authorities experienced difficulties obtaining and interpreting information aimed at addressing need, examining financial commitments, and ensuring information systems fed into each other.[234] Economists believe that the Achilles heel of marketing is quality. Academics on the other hand suggested that for a quasi-market philosophy to be successful there must be large numbers both of providers and of purchasers.

Guidance for social service departments suggested there should be different types of contracts to reflect the different relationships between the various providers. Howard Glennerster and Jane Lewis (1996)[235] discovered what in fact happened was variations on service agreements and contracts. The introduction of the brokerage service with block and spot contracts all added to the creation of a new culture of social care for social service departments. Most authorities began by using spot contracts; this was apart from the commitment already in place for in-house block contracts. However, for practical reasons associated with administration and staffing costs, and ensuring supply, there was soon a move towards the more cost-effective block contracting.[236] A problem soon identified with block contracts was the tendency to simply replace the local authority as provider with an independent organisation and this became known as the *set list syndrome*.[237] Block contracts failed service users in the sense that they did not improve choice and were not flexible. For example, a block contract with a residential home for a total period of five years is highly inflexible. Monitoring contracts, therefore, became a crucial part of the overall contracting process, and the experience in the United States demonstrated that this was one of the most problematic areas. Penalty points and users satisfaction consultations all had their problems.

MODERNISING SOCIAL SERVICES THROUGH BEST VALUE

Another innovation introduced by the Conservative government was compulsory competitive tendering – CCT – which allowed councils to put out to tender, to the private sector, services that historically had been managed and run by the local authority. The government suggested most local authority services were suitable for compulsory competitive tendering, with the exception of services below a certain 'value'. To some degree this gave councils control over which parts of the service they put forward and which they chose not to, although with the introduction of community care the expectation had been for local authorities to contract out most services to independent providers.

When the Labour administration was elected in 1997, it replaced CCT with *Best Value*. During the early stages of Best Value, the government published a set of principles, which outlined what Best Value would mean in terms of strategic planning and service delivery. In the consultation paper

Modernising Local Government: Improving Local Services through Best Value, published in 1998,[238] a number of key steps were identified as necessary to implement the process.

Key steps

Corporate overview

> *Key Step i:* a corporate view of what an authority wants to achieve and how it performs, measured against key indicators and the aspirations of the local community.[239]

The government wanted a new approach that underpinned service provision right across the council's activities and involving all services. Best Value would be more flexible and responsive to the needs of the local community. At the heart of this initiative was a concern to reinvigorate local government with the objective of increasing efficiency in services.

Service planning and service reviews

> *Key Step ii:* an agreed programme of fundamental performance reviews, with a presumption that it will look at areas where performance is worst, and complete a full cycle of reviews over a 4/5 year period.[240]

The government proposed that local authorities should carry out *performance reviews*. These reviews could take the form of investigating a particular geographical area or a social group such as learning disabilities. In line with community care legislation, social service departments were required to produce three-year plans for consulting service users, their families and carers. In addition they were asked to take an active role in the co-ordination of and contribution to joint planning through the joint consultative machinery.

> *Key Step iii:* fundamental performance reviews, each of which challenge the purpose of a service or group of services, compare the authority's performance with others, consult the community, and provide for competition where appropriate.[241]

However, the difficulty was that there exists a tension between central and local government with service indicators and performance targets. The problem was one of nationally set standards weighed against the freedom many local authorities argue should be their right for consulting with the local community. Councils believe that exercises which discuss the standard of services locally assist the local community to make informed choices.

Benchmarking

Benchmarking as a method for reviewing services, incorporates a variety of sources such as official government monitoring returns, inter-borough working groups and commissioned research. The Audit Commission and the Social Services Inspectorate have played an increasingly important part in monitoring progress on performance improvements.[242] These organisations, through the joint review process, have assisted local authorities to contribute to policy development, benchmarking and strategic planning. The Audit Commission outlines its role:

> The Audit Commission is clearly going to have a strategic role in promoting and monitoring benchmarking and performance on these issues. Too often in the past, local authority departments have found that the balance between standards and quality on the one hand and efficiency and economy on the other has not been maintained by reliance on purely audit mechanisms. Attention has been focused on efficiency and economy largely because these are easier to quantify and measure.[243]

Improving performance

> *Key Step iv:* the setting of targets for improved performance and efficiency, together with clear identification about how these improvements are to be achieved, and published in local performance plans.[244]

Best Value not only seeks to be a cost-effective enterprise but it also aims to establish a culture of continuous improvement in light of what communities want from services. In principle, therefore, the initiative has been based upon neutrality from those who provide the service. What distinguishes Best Value is the framework within which it operates aiming to ensure there is no duplication in service provision. The approach characterised by CCT was one of inflexibility with no room for partnership working. The Labour government recognised this fact, and said it wanted Best Value to develop 'relationships based on trust and co-operation rather than the antagonistic relationships that contracts under CCT often gave rise to'.[245] Instead Best Value sought to build on existing requirements under community care legislation with the emphasis on local consultation and user participation. Consultation would include service users, local taxpayers and the wider business community, investigating existing services and discovering ways to meet future needs. One criticism levelled at Best Value has been that it has not called for local authorities to consult their own workforce. Staff working within local government not only have invaluable knowledge about service delivery and gaps in services, but many have first-hand experience of involving users in decisions about their services. In particular, front-line staff, such as keyworkers, often have the confidence and trust of some of the most vulnerable and excluded citizens. Not taking advantage of this knowledge has been a loss to local authorities for gaining a comprehensive picture of the opinions and views of a wide cross-section of the public.[246] The government argued that its approach to Best Value was not based on ideology, but rather was firmly rooted in the phrase 'what matters is what works'.

CONSULTATION AND BEST VALUE

Best Value is concerned with improving public services and providing high-quality services that can be measured. The initiative seeks to ensure that services are delivered in the best possible way, and that they are continually improved through performance monitoring. Since the introduction of Best Value, the government has required local authorities to improve accountability, cost-effectiveness and efficiency of the services provided to local people. *Valuing People* states that at the heart of the government's proposals for people with learning disabilities is for them to gain from services, both mainstream and specialist, and to ensure this happens, resource allocation must be seen in the context of the likely increase in demand for services. The White Paper observes that in certain cases money, currently spent on services to people with learning disabilities, could be used more effectively, arguing that the application of Best Value principles will achieve better value for money.[247]

Quality assurance systems and performance management indicators for learning disabilities services are undeveloped, and other areas of services to people with learning disabilities neglected include complaints, often an effective method for monitoring the success or failure rate of services. In *Valuing People* the government states that the complaints process is in many cases inaccessible to people with learning disabilities, and is complex and difficult for them to understand.

Service planning, policy development and standard setting are all key areas of Best Value. The initiative has taken over the lead in this area from the community care reforms, seeing needs-led services as the foundation of the care in the community philosophy. Bransbury[248] makes a valid point about the attitude of local authorities towards user empowerment by questioning whether:

> ... social services departments, required to contain expenditure on community care, could ever deliver on the promise of 'needs-led' services, whatever structures and processes were in place ... [and this is a question] equally relevant to best value.[249]

This is not to suggest that tight budget restrictions should be used as a reason for not involving service users in consultation. The challenge for Best

Value is finding ways of offering realistic choices to those involved in consultation. Best Value will need to develop ways of managing the problems between available budgets and the public's reasonable expectations for services.[250]

A commitment to change

Best Value seeks to change services and make them accessible to the community as a whole. A commitment to social inclusion, consultation and participation is ultimately a commitment to change. Change is a frightening process for all involved, both for people with learning disabilities, who often prefer familiar surroundings and known situations, and for the professionals attempting to implement the changes. An illustration of this is when day centres have attempted a move towards new and more innovatory schemes, such as training and paid employment outside the centre. This has resulted in uncertainty about the future, and confusion about what the other alternatives offered may represent. Studies have highlighted that what happens in many cases is a *'save our centre'* campaign instigated by what are seen as defensive parents, carers and users voicing their resistance to any changes.[251] Supporters of change have argued that the fear change can cause is an important lesson to be learnt. People with learning disabilities are less likely to be worried if they are presented with a clear vision for the future that also highlights their part in planning their own services. Consultation has a valuable place in the strategic vision and management of successful change.[252] A good consultation strategy should examine the dynamics surrounding the power relationships between professionals and users, and suggest new methods that will allow clearer communication between both groups at an individual level and a structural one. An essential element of the design for a participation and inclusion strategy is the commitment to taking a democratic approach to services. Rob Grieg, addressing a conference on the Foundation for People with Learning Disabilities, points out that change rarely takes place overnight. He draws the following conclusions:

> 'We need to change the culture, the way we think, otherwise service changes will fall apart rapidly. The White Paper is about making a new start in the relationship between statutory sector services and family carers – the language used in this relationship is often the language of war, we need to change this.'[253]

There is a difficulty, however, when consultation becomes incorporated into a process where decisions have already been taken, but masquerades as a democratic exercise. The range of problems for consultation is difficult to resolve; such as, while changes proposed may suit some, not everyone will be in agreement. Parents and carers have over the years been encouraged to speak on behalf of their sons and daughters, brothers and sisters, but this has led to tensions around user participation because of the attitude both of parents and of professionals which is one of "we know what is best".[254] With the changing nature of participation and the shift in emphasis away from the parents speaking on behalf of their children, it has been important for the role of the parents and carers not to be devalued and for their contribution not to be lessened.

Best value and cultural diversity

People with learning disabilities do not constitute a homogenous group, and a related but equally important area of the debate around user consultation is that of recognising the diversity that exists among them. It is a fact that some groups are almost exclusively under-represented in services.[255] Professionals involved in service planning have realised at a very early stage that the issue of equality of access posed questions and dilemmas that often do not have an obvious or right answer. Some difficulties needing to be taken into account when examining equity are:

- service users come from very different backgrounds;
- they will have had very different past experiences;
- their strengths and capabilities will vary;
- they will have a range of different beliefs and values.[256]

The Best Value initiative implies that serious account has to be taken of culture. However, in doing so, professionals are likely to be challenged by problems which may arise when what is acceptable within a particular culture may be regarded as inappropriate in the context of mainstream ideas, for example, sexism or racism. To what extent, for example, is it appropriate to impose mainstream western values on people from different cultures who find them quite alien? Such questions raise serious concerns with no simple easy answer or quick-fix solutions. Most professionals say they try to work out what is the most appropriate course to follow with each particular situation, but professionals need to be mindful of the fact that

> By implication, participation is *not* just about involving people with learning difficulties in the immediate provision of specialist services, but also enabling them to have a wider voice and to influence organisations which can affect their *lives*. Therefore, any participation strategy needs to be outward looking, with efforts made to ensure that policy makers in the wider framework are made aware of the impact of their decisions on people with learning difficulties.[257]

It has been argued that consultation is not about a transfer of power from professionals to users, their parents and carers, but it is about sharing experiences of life, insights and knowledge between a group of people with a collective experience.²⁵⁸ Ghazala Mir, co-author of the report on learning difficulties and minority ethnic communities that accompanied the White Paper, points to the serious lack of knowledge and low levels of take-up of services within the ethnic communities, saying:

> If services are to reach people then they must use the networks that are already there within the ethnic minority communities – not just the structures that services have always used.²⁵⁹

NOTES

225 Howard Glennerster, Anne Power and Tony Travers, 'A New Era for Social Policy: A New Enlightenment or a New Leviathan?', STICERD working paper 39 (London: London School of Economics, 1989).

226 Jane Lewis, 'Purchaser/Provider Splits in Social Care: Context and Issues', in *The Future of Social Services? Lessons for Best Value from the Purchaser/Provider Split*, (ed.), Lynda Bransbury (London: Local Government Unit, no year given).

227 ibid., p. 14.

228 Howard Glennerster and Jane Lewis, *Implementing the New Community Care* (Buckingham: Open University Press, 1996).

229 Lewis, 'Purchaser/Provider Splits', p. 15.

230 Howard Glennerster and Julian Le Grand 'The Development of Quasi Markets', in 'Welfare Provision in the United Kingdom', *International Journal of Health Services* (1995) 25, no. 2: 203–18.

231 Lewis, 'Purchaser/Provider Splits', p. 15.

232 Department of Health and Social Services Inspectorate, *Purchase of Services Guidance* (London: HMSO, 1991).

233 R. Gutch, *Contracting Lessons from the US* (London: National Council of Voluntary Organisations [NCVO], 1992).

234 V. Bovell, J. Lewis and F. Wookey 'The Implications for Social Services Departments of the Information Tasks in the Social Care Market', *Health and Social Care in the Community 5*, no. 2 (London: 1997): 94–105.

235 Glennerster and Lewis, *Implementing*, p. 17.

236 M. Macintosh, 'Flexible Contracting? Economics Cultures and Implicit Contracts in Social Care Partnership' (Buckingham: Open University, unpublished paper).

237 J. Baldock and C. Ungerson, *Becoming Consumers of Community Care* (York: Joseph Rowntree Foundation, 1994). Hoyes and Harrison. L. R. Lart, R. Means, and M. Taylor, *Community Care in Transition* (York: Joseph Rowntree Foundation, 1994).

238 Department of Environment, Transport and the Regions, *Modernising Local Government: Improving Local Services through Best Value*. (London: HMSO, 1998).

239 David Spencer, 'Some Implications of the Best Value Regime', in *The Future of Social Services? Lessons for Best Value from the Purchaser/Provider Split*, (ed.), Lynda Bransbury (London: Local Government Unit [year no given]), p. 40.

240 ibid., p. 41.

241 ibid.

242 ibid., p. 42.
243 ibid.
244 ibid.
245 ibid.
246 Lynda Bransbury, 'The Right Model for Delivering Social Services?', in *The Future of Social Services? Lessons for Best Value from the Purchaser/Provider Split,* (ed.) Lynda Bransbury (London: Local Government Unit, [year not given]), p. 7.
247 Department of Health, *Valuing People,* p. 95.
248 The Bransbury article omits the year of publication.
249 ibid., p. 6.
250 ibid., pp. 6–7.
251 This will become an area for much debate as the principles that *Valuing People* proposes for the future of services become clearer. The government is committed to modernising and improving day services over a five-year period, with the aim of enabling service users to have full and purposeful lives by developing links with employment services and community education. Partnership Boards are required to develop strategic plans for a modernisation programme; however, the modernisation agenda must be in a position to offer greater flexibility and choice.
252 Ken Simons, *A Place at the Table? Involving People with Learning Difficulties in Purchasing and Commissioning Services* (Plymouth: British Institute for Learning Difficulties [BILD], 1999), p. 14.
253 Internet: 'Local concerns for learning difficulty white paper aims' (May 3 2001): http://www.community-are.co.uk
254 Simons, *A Place at the Table?,* p. 23.
255 E. Emerson and C. Hatton, 'Residential Provision for People with Intellectual Disabilities in England, Wales and Scotland', *Journal of Applied Research in Intellectual Disabilities* (1998) 11, no. 1: 1–14.
256 Simons, *A Place at the Table?,* p. 10.
257 ibid., pp. 11–12.
258 G. Grant, 'Consulting to Involve, or Consulting to Empower', in P. Ramcharan, G. Roberts, G. Grant and J. Borland (eds), *Empowerment in Everyday Life* (London: Jessica Kingsley, 1997).
259 Internet: 'Local concerns for learning difficulty white paper aims': http://www.community-are.co.uk

5   The local authority's interpretation of government strategies

THE AUTHORITY'S APPROACH TO BEST VALUE

The social service department whose services provide the basis for the investigation of this study, was chosen by the government to be one of the original councils to pilot Best Value. During the first year 1998/9, the council reviewed 15 different services, representing 26 per cent of the department's overall budget spend. The council chose the services for a variety of reasons; some were already improving; others were considered to be failing; yet others were included because they were seen as potential growth areas especially in terms of partnership working between health and social services.

The government extended this programme in March 2000 to include all local authorities, requiring them to review all services over a five-year cycle. Councils were asked to:

Challenge	why services are provided in the way they are.
Compare	their performance against other similar providers.
Consult	service users and the local community about services.
Decide	if someone else could provide that service more competitively.

As a pilot council testing Best Value, the aim was to become a leading local authority that provided: 'high-quality services, delivered on time, in a polite and friendly manner'. The council sought to ensure that the services it offered were efficient, and cost-effective. To ensure that the services were meeting the needs of their service users, the council set up a consultation meeting inviting members of the public to have a say on the proposals for service development, while also pledging to undertake surveys of local residents once every two years. The information gathered would be used to improve services in line with the wishes and choices of the local community. A *Citizens' Panel* was established and in 1999, managers proudly announced that the panel had 1,500 residents across the borough. The professionals continued with this story of success by assuring the local community that the panel would consult regularly on important decisions about the future of social services and other related policy matters.

The council's community care plan was produced as a three-year strategic vision, developed together with local voluntary agencies. Using Best Value the council sought to offer support through a network of systems that included: home helps, day and residential care, meals on wheels, and other specialist assistance such as transport. Most services were provided directly by the social services department but others, controversially, were bought in from outside agencies. The council argued that this mix would ensure services were tailored to meet different needs, and enable vulnerable people to remain active members of their local community. To achieve this the council set itself a number of goals:

- make it simple for people to gain access to services, whether they want to use one or several;
- help prevent problems occurring, rather than simply dealing with them once they have arisen;
- help to protect and empower disadvantaged citizens.

Angela is a planning manager in the learning disabilities department. In the following discussion she speaks about the importance of the community care plans as forming the heart of user consultation. Angela talks about budget constraints seeing them as the main problem restricting choices rather than a lack of consultation. What was interesting about this response from a planning manager was that, as we shall see, it took place at a time when a couple of days earlier, the council had been exposed in the local press as one that failed to consult users about significant planned changes to services.

'The community care plan which we produce in this department is an important part of social services, and consulting on the community care plan is a very important aspect of what we do here. This year we needed to involve the users prior to writing the plan, to get their views. Once this had been done we did a draft of the plan and took it back to a strategic level. The mechanisms for consulting are evolving all the time. For instance when we wrote the last community care plan in 1999, we spent a day with our users looking at the issues around health. We had done some research with the joint health and social service teams prior to asking the views of users. We then followed this with a second day looking at the community care plan. Health staff set about this task with group working, we had a facilitator and used pictures and simple language; from there we began to form the basis of the plan. The draft plan was then sent out to users with pictures. We asked providers, people like Octa and day centre staff, to go through the plan with the clients using the pictures. We also asked for questions using a

facilitator and small user groups. Finally, we produced a document arising from this process. Feedback was not so good in the sense that things
didn't tie up and come together as we had hoped. They wanted a rolling
programme on issues to do with services. When we write the next plan
we will have clearer ideas, even about the process. There will be a specific piece of work such as a day service review, looking at the whole
day service provision right across the borough in-house and external
providers. We have other mechanisms; working with user groups, individual care assessment which care managers already do as part of their
job. We are talking about getting video facilities so that users can have
their views taped and sent into the department. We want to set up a
quality group, and let people know their views are important and they
do have an impact on services, the way their services are shaped. The
department wants to know what people want and that's why we try
and involve them in planning their services. I know it's politically very
trendy at the moment but that's not my personal reason for doing it.
We are struggling in the department.

There is a difficulty in terms of the community care plan. We do
have some givens such as a limited budget that is tied into existing
services and already directed and agreed from on high. Some things
we just can't do. We can't get more staff. It is very clear there isn't any
money for more staff. We are asking opinions and genuinely want to
know, but there are barriers in the department at the moment we are
working in a climate where we have to find 20 per cent savings from
the services provided to people with learning disabilities. Part of what
we talk about in our groups is whatever we do in life we have limited
choices.'

The council provides services to people with learning disabilities, a large
proportion of whom have additional needs such as physical disabilities,
dual diagnosis (mental health and learning disabilities) and autism. The
learning disabilities teams during the first two years of Best Value met all
the targets for assessment, review and care plans set by the department. The
council's promises to people with learning disabilities, 1999–2002, were set
out in the *Best Value Performance Plan 1999* and included:

- opening a new day centre and a new challenging behaviour unit;
- undertaking a review of day opportunities;
- developing the role of the community support team in anticipation of
  its new assessment and treatment service currently being developed by
  the Community Health Trust for people with learning disabilities who
  were also dual diagnosis;
- completing re-commissioning of the borough's largest provider of 24
  hour care;
- supported living schemes.

Other aims set out in the plan were:

- to enable user forums to meet regularly. These were seen as an important way for future services to be developed;
- working towards more integrated services through partnership working;
- completing the first phase of implementing the innovative *Centre for Independent Living,* a new project that gives disabled people themselves control over developing and managing their services;
- providing advocacy sessions;
- consulting carefully and taking people's views into account.

The council attempted to measure how well it performed against a number of *Performance Indicators* or *PIs.* Some of these PIs were set at a national level by the government or the Audit Commission for all councils, while others the council developed ifself. These measures of success sought to demonstrate how well the authority was doing each year, and if services were improving as a direct response to the choices of those who used them. Services were measured and compared at a local level to reflect national performance with other authorities throughout the country.

The Best Value initiative has been based on the idea of 'quasi-market-testing' of services, modelled on the private business sector. Adopting a public sector model was bound to create serious problems for local authorities, because of the significant differences that exist between public and private practice. Local authorities, for example, can never compete with the private sector purely measured on a cost basis. The danger is that local authority services would be provided according to a cost-driven bottom-line basis alone rather than based on choice and user satisfaction. The reality of the initiative therefore may yet prove to be one of increased financial constraints with less user involvement and choice.

Service brokerage

The ethos of the changes which began in the 1980s took the form of mediating structures between the service users, the services they wanted, the professionals and cost. One of the most fundamental steps taken was the transformation of the social worker to care manager, and was a reflection of the new culture of social care which had its roots in the Thatcher ideology for increased efficiency. One objective was to co-ordinate existing services, but the underlying aim for the government was really about saving money. These changes created difficulties almost immediately, because care managers were part of the social services system and as such were not neutral funders of services. They were not required to align themselves to the choices of users, rather their priority was to work within the budget set by the department.[260] Many senior managers welcomed the new care management system, arguing that it had positive aspects compared with the old-style social work system. For example, services could be more closely co-ordinated, while at the same time more consideration was given to the needs and choices of the user. They argued these initiatives led to improved economic efficiency, both in terms of cost and quality. Most families, user groups and advocates, however, did not agree with this, citing a number of reasons why, including the fact that services continued to remain unresponsive and inadequate; and they began to seek a more responsive and sympathetic approach. Criticism had been levelled at local authorities for their failure to plan and develop new and interesting models that were independent of *'the system'* and offered greater user participation. In light of such criticism local authorities looked for new infrastructures they could adopt and decided to develop *Service brokerage*.

Service brokerage had been established as a neutral facilitation between the service user and those providing the services, and was first introduced as a specialist service for people with learning disabilities in British Columbia, Canada, during the 1970s. The Canadian model offered clear aims for the relationship between the broker and the service user in that the broker acted as someone who:

- emphasises the right of the persons with learning disabilities to choose the type of services they want to meet their needs.
- assists the individuals to negotiate funding.
- was independent from the funding agency and the provider agency.[261]

The broker's role was that of an *agent* with a thorough knowledge of the social care market and with an expertise in their user group. Brokerage has a number of main functions including: identifying services; negotiating funding; implementing and monitoring contractual agreements with community service systems and individual service providers.[262]

In theory, the neutrality of the brokerage system avoids any possibility for a conflict of interest. It provides a single point of entry for accessing a range of services, and in this way the user is not simply expected to take what's on offer. Many critics of the system point out that the original design for brokerage was to empower families to take control, and brokerage was a neutral service. However, when social service departments adopted the model, brokerage lost the independent status it had, because brokers were employed by the council. It was no longer the Canadian model and with time brokerage within many local authorities now incorporates a number of additional functions such as contracting, becoming more business-like in the approach to social care.

The learning disabilities section of the council under investigation was one of the first social services departments in this country to introduce a brokerage service. David has worked as a broker in the learning disabilities department since the service began there in 1996. He spoke about how brokerage operated, and this example shows just how different from the original Canadian model brokerage has become.

'Basically we are responsible for negotiating contracts and costs for the care manager, residential services, respite, that sort of thing. One of the ideas is for costs to decrease as the user becomes more independent. The person needs less support and we monitor that process through the reviews. As a broker, I have virtually no contact with the user. There is no relationship with them, because that's the job of the care manager, OTs and other people who work closely with them. Those are the people who consult with the user and their advocate. We just set up the service. We carry out a brokerage review once a year where we do visit the residential home and meet with the client to find out if they are happy with the placement and the service. If the client says they aren't happy then we tell them to talk it over with the care manager. We just talk to the client and say: "What's it like here?" That's about it. We don't concern ourselves with choice, that's not for us to do. In a nutshell we don't have any contact with the client.'

Andrea is a broker working alongside David. She had previously been a broker for another social services department working for older people services. Her approach to user involvement and brokerage differs somewhat from that of David.

'It's no good seeing our users as just a group of people with generic needs. We have a specific contract with individual headings aimed to meet their needs. We are trying hard to move towards involving service users and letting them have a hand in the contract process. At the moment we are only working with a small group. We may even just pick a user so that there is some representation, some voice. I suppose the big question for brokerage has to be who do you involve and why? For example, I can write a service specification and draw up a contract for one home that can accommodate twenty people, that's where the difficulty is and why I talk about voice and representation. Twenty people have twenty different sets of needs. There is another question and it's about the ability and confidence of the user to communicate. A high percentage cannot become involved in the process because of these barriers. None of us I think fail to recognise these as real issues. The choices are identified through the care manager that is the framework. Brokers communicate with the care managers.'

Many support the brokerage service with accountability to the user. They point to lessons which can be learnt from past mistakes. In the past, for example, professionals were not accountable to the individual, but some attempts have been made to redress this with the introduction in 1993 of devolved budgets, when departments were split into purchasers, headed by a commissioner, with a separate provider department.[263] These structures were as a direct response to the Griffiths recommendations, and sought to allow a greater degree of choice for the 'consumer'. However, Peck and Smith in their 1989 study 'Safeguarding Service Users'[264] highlight the conflicting roles where the assessor of need and the budget gatekeeper are mixed. They argue this creates a serious disincentive to meeting needs, with the problem becoming even more concentrated because most of the devolution takes place *within* social services departments. The only true way for the customer to have choice and flexibility over his or her services, is not through a brokerage system, but by giving funding directly to the users. Writers such as Salisbury *et al.* (1987) note that:

> The most compelling way to ensure system flexibility, responsiveness and accountability is for the government to allocate funding to the person served rather than to programs, services or agencies.[265]

With the publication of *Valuing People* has come the introduction of direct payments to people with learning disabilities, which may change considerably the role of the broker. David reported on his views of the future direction of brokerage:

> 'The future is bright for brokerage. I feel the use of brokerage is going to increase as more is privatised and externalised, the service will need to increase. The government are giving more and more emphasis to recording things like they have done with Best Value. They are looking at more ways of monitoring, performance indicators, that sort of thing.'

Andrea was similarly optimistic about the future:

> 'As long as there is a role for care managers there will be a role for brokers. With the coming together of health and social services staff, brokerage will flourish. It will be essential for a co-ordinated purchasing strategy to be in place.'

Direct payments

In April 1997, social service departments were given the power by the government to provide cash to the disabled for assistance. Direct payments were introduced to empower disabled people to have choice and control over how their support needs were met, and to give them financial independence. In the original government legislation all service user groups were included with the exception of people with learning disabilities. The legislation has moved on since then and people with learning disabilities are now included, but the problems surrounding the whole issue of direct payments to people with learning disabilities are fraught with difficulties because of the emphasis on users as administrators and employers.[266] For the majority of people with learning disabilities it was thought that they were not capable of taking the responsibility for employing their own carers, and this was reinforced through the early legislation which stated that individuals must be able to consent to direct payments. Because of this difficulty a number of independent schemes were set up offering their own advice, training and consultancy initiatives. A report produced by Values into Action in 1997, for example, lists a number of organisations that have chosen this route including the National Centre for Independent Living.[267]

Putting the purchasing control into the hands of service users had the potential for revolutionising social care, allowing people to have the services they wanted, delivered where they wanted, enabling them to lead the type of life they wanted. To a large extent the success of this scheme depends on who has the ultimate control over funding, and in principle it appears straightforward: instead of public money being given to an agency, it is given directly to the individual. However, among some of the potential complications for direct payments are:

- ensuring taxpayers' money is used appropriately;
- making sure there is a system in place whereby funds are shared equitably between those who need them;
- the need for a monitoring system to show funds are being spent in an appropriate way;
- an agreement on the part of the user (or their agent) to take on the responsibility for buying their own support;
- a system allowing for flexibility so that moneys can be changed quickly according to the person's changing needs.[268]

How best to develop user control and hand funding to disabled individuals is an area that has been investigated in Great Britain, since as early as the mid-1940s. Until recently the law in England and Wales prohibited local authorities from making direct payments to people. It was for this reason that a third party organisation was established which would receive the funding and pass it on to the disabled person. An example of this practice can be seen with the *Independent Living Fund* (ILF) set up in 1988. This was a pot of money that was not connected to either social security or social services, and one to which disabled people could apply in order to live an independent life. However, the demand was so great for this type of funding that the budget soon reached levels that were politically unacceptable. Because of this the ILF regulations were revised in 1993, and linked to both social security and social service structures. A significant change came in 1996 with the introduction of the Community Care (Direct Payments) Act.[269] The Act removed the legal block on local authorities, allowing them to make payments directly to the individual if they wished. They were encouraged to do this but not obliged to do so.

Many early innovations for successfully changing the way services were funded, can be attributed to one major reason: the disabled people fighting for change were articulate, assertive and determined to make change happen. Although this was a positive step forward it also had a negative impact in the sense that it led to the assumption that only people with the ability to manage funding themselves could benefit from direct payments. Where an individual had profound learning disabilities, the funding was allocated to a parent, guardian or other agent. In some cases contracts were established between the user and funder, built into which were terms of agreement, monitoring procedures, and an outline of the services to be provided.[270] Some Independent Living schemes run by local authorities allocated money directly to users with physical disabilities. Other users preferred not to administer the funds directly, but still wished to retain control over whom they hired. Stainton (1994) sees several difficulties arising from an individualised funding system and observes:

> It is important to note that individualised funding does not refer to mechanisms which simply allocate a block of funds to a purpose if there is no specific reference to the individuals' needs. For example, a standard per diem grant to a residential service can only be considered "individualised" in the weakest sense, since it is based on a "class" conception of needs and the providers' average costs. This type of funding provides an incentive for agencies to "cream", or to take those persons whose net cost to the organisation is lowest. Hence we see a situation where those with more complex needs are left in institutions, or at home with families with no support.[271]

Valuing People is the first White Paper seriously to examine making available direct payments to people with learning disabilities. It states that:

> Promoting direct payments is a key element of our new vision for people with learning disabilities [and] we are extending eligibility for direct payments through legislation.[272]

The Carers and Disabled Children Act 2000 and the Health and Social Care Act 2001 provided scope for direct payments to be extended. Both:

- require local councils to make direct payments where an individual who requests and consents to one meets the criteria;
- enable local councils to make direct payments to the parents of disabled children to meet the child's needs and for local council-provided rehabilitation services.[273]

However, *Valuing People* states that direct payments are an effective way of empowering people with learning disabilities to take control of their lives and extend choice. The Health and Social Care Bill is specifically designed to give people with learning disabilities access to direct payments. *Valuing People* admits that:

> The success of direct payments for people with learning disabilities depends on good support services . . . Schemes must be accessible to people with learning disabilities, so that they too have the right support to manage a direct payment and remain in control. Our proposals for developing and expanding advocacy services will enable more people to access direct payments.[274]

It is notable that once again here is a policy, like many in the past, which fails to consider how direct payments to people with cognitive and communication difficulties are to be administered. Even though *Valuing People* talks extensively about direct payments to those with learning disabilities, it fails in terms of social policy to produce a persuasive argument about how this will work in practice. David considered direct payments and the involvement of brokerage:[275]

> 'In this council no service users are receiving direct payments at the moment in learning disabilities. I have heard some care managers are attending workshops and conferences to keep up to date on what's going on. Direct payments are being paid to other groups but not learning disabilities. I think there is a lot of doubt about people with learning disabilities being capable of handling finances. I don't think brokerage will have much involvement with direct payments, it will be care managers working with their users, trying to advise them. Brokers would only get involved if we were asked to draw up a contract, but we wouldn't be advising the user about direct payments. We would continue to provide information to the users on services which are available, daycare, outreach, residential accommodation, inspection and costs. I suppose you could have a system where there wouldn't be the need for brokerage only as an information system, and then that could be dwindled down to a provider file system.'

Andrea had similar doubts:

> 'I can't really imagine direct payments changing much about brokerage, I mean we will still have to identify appropriate service providers.'

Safeguarding the brokerage system

The government does not intend direct payments to replace other funding mechanisms, but direct funding can be used to specifically target the choices of each individual. Core funding for essential need would continue to be concentrated in social service departments with brokerage maintaining a 'fixed point of response'.[276] A further problem for individual funding is accountability and the specific tracking of moneys; who spends what and on what? Effective safeguards such as external auditing needed to be put in place, as the system developed, but in a way that would allow the person to have control over his or her funds. When brokerage, individualised funding, and personal support all work together they create a synergistic effect with each strengthening the other. Central to this network is the user making decisions and choices about her or his services.

The question of the independence of brokerage in the future is crucial, and this is why there is a strong argument for brokerage to be taken away from local authority control and placed with a voluntary body. Voluntary bodies generally operate several safeguards to ensure independence, including, for example, management committees, whereas the private sector tends not to have such stringent checks. For many commentators the voluntary sector would be the preferred option, because there is no likelihood of profit being a motivating force. Brokerage and individual funding create the opportunity for more flexible and responsive services, but how these are co-ordinated still remains an unanswered question. Those in favour of the brokerage system point out that it provides an effective method for service planning, because it acts as an information system keeping an up-to-date record of services to which both users and staff can have access.[277] This information can also give a clearer indication of community needs with priority services more easily identified. However, a contentious issue for services remains one of cost and although brokerage is in its infancy as a service in Britain, the initial results from research suggest that having a brokerage system can substantially reduce cost over time. It is argued brokerage offers a cohesive method for uniting the demands of the individual with innovations in social policy practice.

THE COUNCIL'S COMMITMENT TO PEOPLE WITH LEARNING DISABILITIES 1999–2002

At the beginning of 1999, there were 547 people with learning disabilities aged 18 and over who were the responsibility of social services, most of whom lived in the borough but some were placed outside. A database was established within the department to store information about individuals with the intention of using the data to plan and develop key services in response to what users were saying they needed. The database held detailed information on people such as their age, ethnicity, additional disabilities, chronic health needs, and the age of any carer(s) involved.

The council examined for this project was one of the first inner London boroughs to establish partnership working between health and social services. In the learning disabilities section, there was a multi-disciplinary team of 55 professionals, providing social and health care services ranging from assessment and care management to specialist health clinicians. These teams were responsible for providing:

- residential homes with 24-hour support;
- adult placements where the client is placed in a carer's own home;
- packages of care provided in the client's own home;
- respite care;
- day centres;
- sheltered work placements;
- open employment.

The council's Community Care Plan 1999–2000 stated that user involvement was still in the early stages. In December 1997, the council carried out a small survey to canvass the views of users and their carers about becoming involved in consultation meetings. The results revealed that users and their carers valued having a say in the future direction and planning of services. Parents said they wanted to become involved but when staff attempted to involve them they met with indifference. Darren, a commissioning manager, explains:

> 'People with learning disabilities and their parents or carers are included when we write the community care plan, because it is their services we are talking about and meeting their needs – what they want. I think a lot of people often have a more optimistic idealistic view about being consulted, but that's less so now. We attempted to hold a focus group and sent out invitations to parents and carers but *no* parents responded.'

Quite a number of parents had many years of experience dealing with professionals and for them it was the professionals who lacked real interest. A significant number talked about how caring the staff used to be years ago, and how nowadays many parents would not attend any meetings or consultation groups. Jane was one such carer who reminisced about how it used to be and spoke about the 'bond of caring' that had existed. As with many other parents and carers Jane said the rapid turnover of staff greatly contributed to the growing gap and mistrust that currently existed between carers and professionals.

> 'Oh years ago it used to be really good. The communication between carers and service users with professionals has diminished over the last ten years. Ten years ago we had our own social worker to take care of all the issues around the user, and a support worker to manage the carer. I think every carer needs supervision at least four times a year, and also courses should be made available to carers: health and safety, food hygiene, lifting and handling and so on. They produce these plans

and talk about involving parents but it's just that – talk. The staff turnover is a real problem. I feel like I am constantly briefing new staff and new teams who get involved. The social worker who had been so good left and it was a mini tragedy for all of us.'

A senior manager from the learning disabilities team visited the day centre to meet with users and two days of talks were held to discuss their concerns about health and social care issues. The department's plan explains that professionals would be consulting with service users, and this would continue with regular consultation forums. The meetings could be used as a way for dictating the strategic direction services would take until a review in 2002. The strategic focus between 1999 and 2002 was for:

- the best possible provision of community care services;
- improved access to generic and specialist health services;
- full participation in the local community for service users;
- *continued involvement of users in planning their services.*

What was not explained was how the council intended to achieve these aims in a climate where financial constraints were becoming even greater due to the pressure Best Value was placing on local authorities to create cost-effective services.

The department's Community Care Plan highlighted from previous consultations that a main problem was people's feelings of isolation. Users and carers said one reason was a lack of facilities such as flexible and reliable transport, which was consistently raised as a serious problem. It was particularly important for people with learning disabilities and their carers who said the lack of transport was a major obstacle. Public transport was not accessible to many people with learning disabilities, for various reasons: their behaviour in public was offered as one example. A lack of access to leisure facilities featured, as did a lack of information about services presented in a way that was clearly and easily understood. An objective of the plan was that people with learning disabilities should be seen as important members of the local community, and would be helped by a number of key options to facilitate social inclusion. For example, one idea was to provide more support workers. However, the lack of available resources was acknowledged as a problem for funding new initiatives. The council said it intended to tackle this problem by setting up a community inclusion strategy, consisting of professionals, parents, carers and users as well as officers from other departments such as leisure, education, housing and the environment.

Involving people with learning disabilities in service planning calls for a degree of articulation and communication competence if they are going to take an active and productive role. No mention was made of specialist provision in the plan for those who could not communicate their need or participate in the decisions being proposed.

Komfort is a service user who spoke about people who did not communicate well in meetings:

> 'We are all dragged along to these meetings from time to time. Sometimes they're good. It is a problem when people can't always be understood, but I think the professionals don't help with their papers. They are bound by ways of doing things that aren't always flexible. I think what most professionals do are based on papers written by other professionals who may not have direct experiences. It's based on research done a long time ago. About what I'm saying is some people come into whatever profession has interested them when they were at university rather than relying on first-hand experiences. They rely on research that might have been done 10, 15 or 20 years ago. First of all research only focuses on a very small number of people in one place. I think if someone comes up with a new idea that doesn't fit into the pattern of things it's ignored or laughed at. That's how I see meetings. Do they meet my choices? It's a difficult question to give a "yes" or "no" to but I think there's an awful lot of heavy stuff to go through and at the end you may not get what service you want.'

The plan suggested users and their carers were already taking an active role in their own assessments and reviews, but it proposed further measures such as more time to allow users, carers and advocates to make comments about assessment procedures and draw up their own contribution to the plan. Care managers had the responsibility for ensuring users' views were included.

The department had a Joint Commissioning Group that set out how it intended to include users and their carers in decisions about the future of their services. It produced a number of strategies including:

- users/carer satisfaction surveys;
- meeting with user/carer groups such as *People First*;
- specific meetings around particular topics;
- *where major changes are to be made consulting users and carers about the need for change, in order that they fully participate in shaping future services*;
- identifying ways to encourage people with learning disabilities from ethnic minority groups to take up services that are culturally appropriate.

The section of the plan that discussed the funding of services opens by saying: 'There is no available new money in the system' and continues 'all the proposals suggested in this plan will come from within existing resources'. The plan acknowledged the problems that additional care placements would encounter in terms of extra funding, which was not available, but went on to say that discussions will be taking place to establish where the extra money can come from. These rather high-flown ambitions need to be seen in the context of the council's targets for departmental budgets for the year 2000–1. The immediate question this raised was whether the council was setting itself up to fail because of elaborate strategic planning and user consultation forums with no money in the pot to fund the development of existing services or potential new ones arising from users' choice? It was not long before this question received unwelcome wider public attention, and the consultation strategy was revealed to be at odds with the rhetoric of the department. The manner in which services were financed and administered by the professionals became a very public debate when, on 21 October 1999, the local press began a series of articles, apparently leaked from within the council. The headlines and opening of the first article read:

RESIDENTS OF CARE HOME FACING PRIVATISATION WERE NOT CONSULTED

A HOME for people with learning difficulties could be turned over to a private company in a bid to claw back £100,000 from the council's social services budget. The social services committee agreed to let officials look into proposals for the home in Westbourne Crescent at a meeting of its sub-committee.

The article continued:

Residents at Westbourne Crescent were present at the meeting but because their carers are council employees no deputation was made. The proposals are part of a raft of suggestions designed to save £200,000 from the social services budget. The Director said learning difficulties services had been targeted because their costs were disproportionately high. "We've been able to reduce costs of some packages by £100,000", he said. "We have a problem with the remaining £100,000 . . . changing care arrangements at the home, which currently houses five people with learning difficulties at a cost of £180,000 a year, would help meet the cuts." "There are alternative providers in the borough who can do this considerably cheaper," he said. No one at the home had, however, been informed about the possibility of turning it over to a private company, Cllr Charles Freeman told the committee. "It's clear that the residents and carers had no notice at all of the existence of this report and I'm very concerned about that", he said.

The Director admitted the home had not been informed of the proposals. "We should have worked with them more and re-assured them", he said.

In another section of the paper on the same day the dramatic headline stated:

GET OUT BY CHRISTMAS EVE

It read:

> A group for people with learning difficulties is being turfed out of its home at Christmas, as cold-hearted Council bosses say they no longer need the building.
>
> A self-help group for people with learning difficulties have been told to vacate their premises by Christmas Eve as the Council is terminating its lease on the building. The Council's lease with the freeholders had stipulated the buildings must be used as offices. But most of the organisations run groups and workshops, and are not strictly offices.
>
> However, the owners have written to the Council saying they support the present use of the building as a "valuable community resource" and would be willing to renew the lease on this basis once it ran out.
>
> But a spokeswoman for the Council said they were unlikely to consider renewing it. "We are terminating the lease as we no longer have a use for the building."
>
> Stephen, a company director, whose company lease space in the building, said they were hoping to put forward a package that would save the present use of the building and be acceptable to the Council. He said, "We are not taking this lying down, we are looking at other ways of maintaining the building as a community resource."
>
> He said it was "totally wrong" to force people with learning difficulties to leave by December. "They do not need to do that, they will not be putting anyone else in that space in the interim."

The political embarrassment experienced by the council continued with the publication of a further article with the banner headline:

FORGOTTEN CLAIM COSTS US £84,000
OFFICIALS WERE TOO BUSY WITH ASYLUM SEEKERS

> BUNGLING Council Officers missed out on an £84,000 government grant because they failed to put the application in on time, social services committee heard.
>
> At the same meeting, Councillors were asked to put Westbourne Crescent home for people with learning difficulties into private hands and consider closing a café which teaches cooking skills to people with learning disabilities because the department needs to make £200,000 worth of cuts to meet its budget.

A Councillor, who spotted the mistake in a report to the audit sub-committee and insisted social services members be told, said he was not happy about the handling of the application.

"They lost £84,000 and it's significantly more than the money they would save from closing the Café", he told the paper.

The claim for the grant, issued by the Department of Health to fund social services training programmes, should have been made to the Council's financial division by the end of September 1998. But in March the Department of Health contacted the Council to find out what had happened to its application. Officers were given until 3 p.m. on March 9 to get the claim in. They failed to meet the deadline and social services will have to make up the shortfall. "The only thing that bucked them up was a fax from the Department of Health and they still couldn't get it in", said the councillor. He thought the claim had been "forgotten" and the mistake had seriously affected this year's budget.

The social services director told councillors he was "mortified" when he discovered the claim had not gone in. He said it was over-looked because officers were dealing with asylum seeker claims which took priority. "I agree it's not acceptable", he said.

The report to the committee said a series of changes in zhandling of grant applications would be made.

The final article in this series appeared leading up to the Christmas period when on 12 December the paper ran the story:

PROTEST OVER HOME TAKEOVER HEATS UP

OPPONENTS of a plan to turn a council home for people with learning difficulties over to a private company have stepped up their campaign to force the Council to rethink.

Residents at the home in Westbourne Crescent, their parents and the Unison representatives plan to lobby the local MP to join their campaign to force the social services committee to reject the cost-cutting measures.

The group fears that residents will suffer and the move could lead to the privatisation of the entire supported living scheme that currently covers ten projects. "There is no justification for these plans", said the Unison representative. "The workforce has shown great loyalty . . . why attack a successful service?"

The Director told the committee in October that residents' needs would be assessed but campaigners say the change could jeopardise the continuity of care they receive and their needs have not been formally evaluated.

This study revealed that the attitude of the majority of parents and carers interviewed saw initiatives such as the community care plan as little more than another unhelpful layer of bureaucracy, designed to hide the real truth – financial constraints. Some were extremely angry at the way in which they had been treated in the past, while others felt resigned to the 'high-handed' authority demonstrated by the professionals and sought help through other, and for them, more powerful avenues.

Robert worked as a policeman for 26 years. His three sons are now grown up. Michael at 37 is the youngest and has Down's Syndrome and autistic tendencies. In 1988, Robert's wife left him. She moved out of the family home to live with another man. Robert was devastated. He found himself with custody of three small children, and a full-time job to hold down. Robert battled to bring up his children on his own. Michael's behaviour from 1988 onwards became increasingly difficult to manage, and Robert turned to social services for help. Robert recounts what happened next:

'I just don't get involved anymore with their meetings, their plans and the like. My wife left us in '88, and I found myself with three young children to bring up. I approached social services. I'm a policeman you see. Anyway I approached social services for help. Have a guess what they said. They told me to give up my job. Being a policeman I was in what is called a "tied" house that's where the house and the job go together. So if I gave up my job I would have to get out of the house. I explained all this to them. Imagine that clever suggestion. They said they could only help if I lost my house and found myself homeless with the kids. What would happen to my children then? They'd be taken straight into care wouldn't they? The only way round it was I worked nights and found care during the day for the children, I paid for that. I phoned social services and asked them to help me with Michael. I was desperate, he's not the easiest to look after at the best of times. They said of course we will help. I was really pleased, tell you the truth I felt such relief. Then they asked how will I pay for it: the cost was £10.00 an hour. I was flabbergasted: you're talking a lot of money. I didn't know what to do. A friend told me about Octa and said I should go there. I approached them and got a live-in carer that I paid for. Initially that was just over a quarter of my income just on this carer. I kept at social services and eventually they picked up the cost.

Social workers, they're very nice people but they're not effective. In my profession, as a policeman, I have often been called out to solve a problem at 2 a.m. in the morning. With social services there is a lot of talk. It's talking, paperwork, reviews and plans. Talking shops all the time, we talk a lot and there isn't any real follow-through. Imagine if the police force behaved like that. They come to this council but they don't stay long. I want Michael to live in full-time residential care, I'm getting older for one thing and the others have left home years ago. I'm not able to cope with Michael; he's autistic as well as having Down's Syndrome – that takes some looking after. I want residential care for him but we've been talking for years.

There's no point going to their meetings, I won't go to meetings. I won't unless there will be a real outcome. There never is, there's never a likely outcome. Too many people have meetings about meetings. They talk about consulting us but what's the point. No decisions are made. This is the way forward and this is how we are going to achieve it – that doesn't happen. I'm not going to a talking shop. It's all budget talk. We meet the social worker, we talk about respite care, they talk about how much it will cost, and we get angry. I raised three kids on my own, I do a harsh job. I don't like to be given the run around. Lovely well-meaning nice young people but they don't have the tools.

Most parents I know wash their hands of the social workers. They come and go but parents, we can't walk away; it's our lives, and they're our children. It destroys your faith when you think something is going to happen and it doesn't. It's especially difficult to deal with when that happens. Parents I know have given up on services because they are not reliable. These days I get services through Octa and they are very good in many ways. It has taken a long time to build up a relationship with them. They teach Michael travel training, he has a tendency to wander, and other skills like cooking and cleaning, but his ability is really very limited.'

Margaret's son Philip is autistic and lives in a residential home run by the council. The problems of bureaucracy and her sense of isolation have their roots in a much wider political agenda between the professionals and councillors. Margaret also highlighted the problems caused by the staff turn-over:

'They talk about consulting parents and have elaborate community plans, but the problems for parents are often more immediate than that. There is a rapid turn-over of staff which is difficult because my son needs a lot of individual attention. With Philip, after a while working with him, staff get discouraged because of his behaviour. The support workers come up with all sorts of things to stimulate him and amuse him, but he loses interest so quickly.

Where social services committee are concerned I think members are well intentioned, but officers are a mixed bunch. It's all part of the chequered history of the home where Philip lives. A few years back we [the parents] heard they couldn't afford to spend money on the home, the home was in a terribly rundown state, and we were left wondering what the motive was. We get very paranoid about motives. There had been various changes about the running of the home. Then I heard Philip was given medication inappropriately. I went to the home and I challenged the manager about it. I got no joy so I went to the senior manager who was head of that section. She told me about the complaints procedure, and I went home that evening feeling happy because I felt I was being listened to. Eventually that manager went and a new one took over. The most recent thing we have been talking about for the home are licensing agreements, which are a bit like a tenancy and gives more security to our children. I understand though that neither the housing department nor the social services department are very serious about this. I don't know if it is because of the intervention of the councillors. We did meet with the housing department, and the borough's legal department, and came up with something I'm hopeful of.

The other thing I want to mention is the liaison group for people with learning difficulties, ever since I heard about it I turn up regularly, because the councillors are involved. You can talk in the open and get some action. I feel with the high-up officers they go into a huddle and decide things and it's the way it's then presented to everyone else. It's a very powerful position. Budgets are tight and sometimes the officers let their own agendas take precedence and to do it under the guise of money well what a splendid idea – you know what I'm talking about! Councillors are in a way members of Parliament they have to take it up when we ask them to. We appreciate their involvement, that's why I shall be sorry if local government changes to that kind of mayor style there's so much talk about. There will be lots of prospects for covering up inefficiency and bad management. I think with the whole consultation process there's a lot of inefficiency there already.'

It is such difficulties as these that reflect at a more general level the limited number of initiatives and studies there have been in this area to support and empower parents and carers to participate.

PARTNERSHIP WORKING

People with learning disabilities have been victims of the past in the sense that during the 19th century and in the early 20th century most did not receive any services at all unless they were incarcerated. From 1959, it was decided that, like everyone else, they should enter hospital only for the purpose of receiving treatment for illness. However, no government was courageous enough to highlight that the money which had been spent by the NHS on this group, from this period onwards should have been handed over to local authority social service departments. Indeed since 1976 substantial efforts have been made in devising strategies to get the NHS to hand over money to local authorities to supply community care services. One question this raises is: 43 years later, why is the NHS still providing services to people with learning disabilities?

Partnership working has set out to make access to services easier for users, but does it aid users to have greater choice over the service they want? Increasingly, the joint health and social care single management structure is being adopted by social service departments throughout Britain. It aims to promote integrated working and, among other things, seeks to establish a more personal and intimate relationship between users and professionals. The following is a definition of partnership working taken from the Department of Health's 1998 document *Partnership in Action (New Opportunities for Joint Working between Health and Social Services)*. It suggests:

> Successful joint working across health and social care will need to be based on shared information and therefore an understanding of what information is required, at both the strategic and operational level, and the establishment of information systems to achieve that is required. At the moment, progress is being held back in many areas by shortcomings in current information systems, by lack of compatibility between health and social care systems and by barriers to the sharing of information.[278]

When community care policy became legislation, assessment of need was seen as the cornerstone. Users became *customers* with the same rights that customers of other services exercised, but the flaw was that these 'customers' function within the constraints of local policy and spending limits, and in this sense could never be consumers with extended choices. The government's answer was to extend consumer choice through the introduction of the purchaser/provider split, which it suggested would result in increased competition, and thus extend quality and choice of services. However, many purchasers and fund holders had little idea about the needs of people with learning disabilities, because of a lack of involvement in their daily lives. Social workers offered GPs as a clear example. In some cases health trusts had become both purchaser and provider, creating an automatic conflict of interests. Powerful and monopolistic trusts could be difficult for purchasers to challenge whatever form they adopted, and partnership working was offered as a solution. Several senior managers within the learning disabilities department, investigated for this study, found monopolistic providers a particular problem. They argued that this ensured users did not gain access to appropriate individually tailored services and choice was limited.[279]

The head of Learning Disability Services spoke about how she attempted to change this situation in partnership with her colleagues in health:

'I see partnership working as part of the greater market philosophy that enables people with learning disabilities [to have] greater choice. In this borough we have made a wonderful example of this philosophy, because we have a major voluntary organisation which is in fact a monopolistic, or monopoly, organisation. It has now grown into a colossal service provider and I would say in fact that it is the major service provider in the borough. Undoubtedly this is disadvantageous for our users because they do not have a choice, or they have severely restricted choices. Do you want me to go on about this, I could get very passionate about it you know? I don't agree with having a service monopoly, because I firmly believe it restricts choice, and so some years ago I set about with other colleagues in health to tender for other organisations to come into the borough and develop new services. A major tendering process began and we now have a second service provider in the borough which is flourishing. It is my intention to continue working with my colleagues in health, because you gain greater insight into the whole needs of those who use our services.'

Elizabeth, another manager, had an equally positive attitude towards the benefits partnership working could achieve. She explained:

'The market theoretically is supposed to respond to choice and partnership practices with health aid this, thus making access to services easier because of a single entry point. Users should have choices in the services they get: where you live, what day service you have, whether you've got a job or not, what support you get so that your needs, if defined adequately, are fully met. There should also be a choice in the styles of providers, and in theory if the market is responding as it is supposed to do, it should ensure that people don't fall outside provision as has historically happened. I think there is a greater danger of this happening if they have more complex needs or are challenging in their behaviour. The theory is that partnership working is in place to meet their whole needs, health and social. I believe the strength of partnership working is the co-ordination of care that it can achieve. I also believe extending choice should mean easier access and this can be done with smaller organisations who are more accessible and less bureaucratic in terms of how people gain access to those services.'

Partnership working revisited

Ward argued in 1995 that serious obstacles needed to be overcome if partnership working was to become a reality. She suggested the NHS & Community Care Act (1990) had specifically negative effects on services for people with learning disabilities, and offered the following key reasons why partnership working would prove to be difficult:

(1) The government did not demand health authorities to hand over money to social service departments, but rather *encouraged* a transfer. Health authorities had from the outset been reluctant to do this. Most of the money raised in the sale of hospitals had been diverted to other areas within the NHS.
(2) There was continuing confusion around some areas as to what constitutes social versus health care and who pays for what.
(3) The policy of community care is filled with rhetoric about user-centred services and choice. The reality is the policy operates within tight budgets.
(4) GPs as fund-holders are often ignorant of the needs of people with learning disabilities and most have limited, if any, contact with community learning disability teams.[280]

For both health and social service authorities there are immediate drawbacks to collaborative working. Organisations do not like to give up their autonomy, and have often sought to remain autonomous minimising any type of dependency on each other. There are difficulties in areas such as the amount of investment of time and energy to develop relationships without any real idea about the possible outcome. The White Paper *Modernising Social Services, Promoting Independence, Improving Protection, Raising Standards,* published by the Department of Health in 1989, argued the aim of community care was to deliver services and reduce boundaries between health and social care. However, research carried out on people with learning disabilities, resettled from long-stay hospitals, suggested progress on partnership working has been slow. Early studies, such as that by Collins in 1992, found that resettlement programmes were often centred on what the hospital staff wanted, rather than the needs or choices of the resident. Another criticism Collins points to was the fact that users were fitted into existing services, rather than having an assessment of need carried out. She also discovered that people were 'prised' out of hospital, many of whom did not want to leave.[281]

Reviewing the extensive literature that exists on community care can only lead to the conclusion that the 1989 White Paper was more optimistic than realistic about partnership working. Webb (1991) is scathing in his criticism:

> ... exhortations to organisations, professionals and other producer interests to work together more closely and effectively [but the reality is] all too often a jumble of services fractionalised by professional, cultural and organisation boundaries and by the tiers of governance.[282]

Webb believes successive governments have refused to recognise the real obstacles which exist to partnership working. Past governments have *requested* social service authorities and health authorities to work together on a range of initiatives, and government has attempted to ensure partnership works by, for example, withholding funding until joint projects have been successfully completed. Inevitably this has not fostered goodwill amongst the agencies, resentment has been the result 'especially where social service departments see health authorities as exploiting unreasonably the pivotal role allocated to them by central government'.[283]

Dalley (1991) suggests three distinct categories where beliefs and behaviour among the different professions cause serious drawbacks to partnership working:

(1) There is a marked difference in professional attitudes to the family, the role of care in the community, and the value placed on institutional care.
(2) Hostility between clinicians and social care professionals was evident and had the effect of strengthening each group's solidarity and identity. Dalley describes this process as 'tribal ties' where professional differences were set within each profession's cultural identity making co-operative working virtually impossible for some authorities.
(3) Managers from health and managers from social services often felt they had more in common with each other (because the demands and pressures of their jobs were similar) than they did with colleagues within the same profession. The same was true of front-line and operational staff.[284]

This final difference may yet add a further complication to undermine partnership working with a growing gap between managers and front-line staff. Front-line staff are often not in a position to comprehend the *wider visions* and decisions taken by senior managers. One way of overcoming this is by developing an operational philosophy on joint working practices with training criteria that would include:

• examining the similarities between the organisations, cultures and values; that would enable collaborative working;
• a shared agreement on roles and responsibilities;
• the value of shared ideas across the organisations, and the problems of alternative resources;
• trust achieved though successful examples of joint working in other areas.[285]

Community learning difficulties teams

In many ways community learning difficulty teams that were set up in the early 1970s, and formerly known as community mental handicap teams

(CMHTs), were the forerunner to partnership working. In the 1970s, they rapidly spread to most parts of the country and demonstrated, albeit to a limited degree, that an inclusive way of working between social services and health authorities could operate successfully. By the 1980s a large number of departments had joint health and social services teams, but this came to an end and they separated with the advent of the purchaser/provider split. However, the size and make-up of these teams had been of interest to researchers. McGrath and Humphreys in their study of *The All Wales Community Mental Handicap Team Survey* in 1988, found that they fell into one of four categories. First, there was a basic type of team that included social workers and users, which in the study equalled 16 per cent. Second, there were larger teams made up of professionally orientated members. Third, there were even larger teams, which this time included all the professionals mentioned before plus service organisers, social workers and nurses. Finally, there were teams that included a cross-section of health and social service professionals. The findings of the research suggested that collaborative working was possible and could be successful. McGrath and Humphreys's research was followed in 1990 by Mansell's study on community learning difficulty teams in Britain. Both studies revealed positive aspects of partnership working that included:

- service planning involved users and carers with practical access to participation;
- clarification of the roles and responsibilities of the professionals involved;
- ways of bringing together all levels of workers right across the spectrum from front-line staff to senior management in health and social services;
- the establishment of professional specialist fieldwork resources.[286]

The government introduced a number of initiatives that it said would help the successful development of inter-agency working. These were laid out in the Department of Health (1999) *Guidance on the Health Act Section 31 Partnership Arrangements*[287] and among the new initiatives introduced was commissioning.

Strategic planning and commissioning

Within the new partnership arrangements, the management of health-related provision for people with learning disabilities was delegated to social services as the lead agency. As lead agency, social services took full responsibility and accountability for the commissioning and integration of services.[288] Two forms of commissioning were introduced: Lead Commissioning and Joint Commissioning. Lead commissioning and joint commissioning are similar and are used countrywide by many local authorities for their learning disabilities services. The Department of Health *Guidance* on commissioning, issued in 1999, stated that lead commissioning provides an effective and efficient way for planning and developing services.[289] However, some health authorities strongly objected to handing over the full responsibility for 'their' services to local authorities because they believed that local authorities did not have a full understanding of health and the clinical expertise to act as lead commissioner from the outset. They preferred instead joint commissioning, which is the process by which two or more commissioning agencies act together to co-ordinate the commissioning of services. Commissioners advise managers and other professionals on the strategic planning of services, and also help to ensure initiatives meet statutory requirements by:

(1) developing a strategic framework for services;
(2) operational planning and purchasing;
(3) reviewing and monitoring services.[290]

The first is about developing services and having a clear vision about how services should work and is the first point at which people with learning disabilities should be involved. The second bears equal importance to the first and is about implementing the department's strategic plans. Finally, reviewing and monitoring is an area that critics suggest has been much neglected in the past;[291] it is about judging what makes a good or bad service, and is an impossible task to carry out without referring to the experiences of service users, their families and carers.

The opportunities that partnership working offers are significant. It aims to increase the quality of services by allowing different professionals to work within a single management structure. Integrated providers include: local authorities, primary care trusts, and NHS trusts ensuring a seamless service. However, the entire concept of partnership working and commissioning is still relatively new and very little research exists examining the long-term effects it may have for including users in service planning.[292] Supporters of partnership working suggest that it counteracts inter-agency conflict, and the initial evidence from authorities who have embarked on this way of working suggests it leads to services developing that are more reflective of the holistic choices and needs of users. The London Learning Disability Strategy Group identified possible strengths and barriers to partnership working including:

Strengths

- more inclusion of users in service planning;
- elimination of inconsistencies in local services – for example, eligibility criteria or the extension of training support across all local services;

- speeding up of decision-making processes;
- increased likelihood of multi-agency and complex projects;
- reduced duplication.

Barriers

- a lack of senior commitment or change in senior management;
- no dedicated time to develop arrangements;
- lack of agreement about aims;
- no clear agreement on service philosophy or service development;
- negative working relationships and a lack of trust amongst key officers and members.[293]

However, to be effective in the sense of reflecting the interests of service users, it may be argued that such strategies require a reasonable level of communication and understanding between professionals and service users. The following chapter seeks to explore the degree of communication evident in other settings in which professionals met service users for the purpose of consultation, and indicates that there might be considerable obstacles to the inclusion of many people with learning disabilities into the planning process.

NOTES

260 S. M. Rose and B. L. Black, *Advocacy and Empowerment* (Boston: Routledge & Kegan Paul, 1985), pp. 74–7.
261 Internet: *"Getting Control of the Money"*: http://www.viauk.org
262 Brian Salisbury, Jo Dickey and Cameron Crawford, *Service Brokerage: Individual Empowerment and Social Service Accountability* (Downsview: G. Allan Roeher Institute, 1987), p. 22.
263 Department of Health, *Implementing Community Care: Purchaser, Commissioner and Provider Roles* (London: HMSO, 1991).
264 Edward Peck and Helen Smith, "Safeguarding Service Users", *Health Service Journal*, 7 December 1989, p. 152.
265 Salisbury *et al.*, *Service Brokerage*, p. 13.
266 Simons, *A Place at the Table?*, p. 73.
267 A. Holman and J. Collins, *Funding Freedom: Direct Payments for People with Learning Difficulties* (London: Values Into Action, 1997).
268 Internet: *"Getting Control of the Money"*: http://www.viauk.org
269 Department of Health, *Direct Payment Act: Policy & Practice* (London: HMSO, 1996).
270 Brian McKenny, "Proposal for Individualized Funding (Draft Three)" (Vancouver: Community Living Society, 1991), pp. 6–10.
271 Stainton, *Autonomy and Social Policy*, 1994 p. 346.
272 Department of Health, *Valuing People*, pp. 48 and 5.
273 ibid., p. 48.
274 ibid.

275 The interviews with David and the other brokers were carried out in 2000, a year before the publication of *Valuing People.*

276 B. McKenny, 'Proposal for Individualized Funding' (Vancover: Community Living Society, 1991), pp. 46–9.

277 Autonomy and Social Policy, 1994, p. 352.

278 Department of Health, *Partnership in Action (New Opportunities for Joint Working between Health and Social Services)*, a discussion document (London: HMSO, 1998), p. 33.

279 J. Collins, *The Resettlement Game* (London: Values Into Action, 1993).

280 Ward, 'Equal Citizens', p. 8.

281 J. Collins, *When the Eagles Fly: A Report on Resettlement of People with Learning Difficulties from Long-stay Institutions* (London: Values Into Action, 1992).

282 A. Webb, 'Co-ordination, a Problem in Public Sector Management', *Policy & Politics* (1991) 19, no. 4: 29–42.

283 R Means and Smith, *Community Care*, p. 141.

284 G. Dalley, 'Beliefs and Behaviour: Professionals and the Policy Process', *Journal of Ageing Studies* (1991): 163–80.

285 B. Hudson, 'Collaboration in Social Welfare: a Framework for Analysis', *Policy & Politics* 15, no. 3 (1987): 175–82.

286 ibid., p. 31.

287 Department of Health, *Guidance on the Health Act Section 31 Partnership Arrangements* (London: HMSO, 1999).

288 ibid., points 34–5.

289 ibid., points 27–9.

290 Simons, *A Place at the Table?*, pp. 5–6.

291 ibid., p. 7.

292 Internet: London Learning Disability Strategy Reference Group: DOH, SSI and NHS: http://www.doh.gov.uk

293 ibid., p. 4.

6　Group observations

It would seem that consultation is a process to which everyone subscribes and the subsequent policies take hours to produce and yet the reports from parents and carers as well as users suggest there are considerable difficulties of communication and distrust from parents who do not find it a helpful exercise to be engaged in. Sometimes service users cannot understand what is going on. Some parents said openly that their children only attend because it represents a day out, nothing more. Quite clearly for many communication is the key problem. Let us have a look at what happens in actual examples of consultation meetings and user participation. How well do the sessions succeed in involving users, parents and carers to have their say, or are they set up to support officers and senior managers who have to carry out the policies? In the following group observations, we shall see that few people with learning disabilities are directly involved, but tremendous reliance is placed on a few 'stars' whom officers, managers and social workers find it easy to communicate with and who are of great importance. Although these star contributors enable a viewpoint to be given, it is difficult to estimate how representative it is. People with learning disabilities, like the rest of society, are a varied group with a range of different interests and needs. Some, for example, agreed with the idea of closing day centres in favour of taking up 'real' jobs in the community, but equally others wanted to stay in the familiar and secure environment of the day centre with the immediate support networks of staff and friends it offered.

OBSERVATIONAL METHODS

The basic task of the participant observer is to observe the people in the group, unit, organisation or whatever is the focus of the enquiry, while being involved with them. Accounts are collected from informants. However, to give form and precision to the data, the observer often has to *ask questions* about the situation and the accounts that are given. These are both questions to oneself, and, more sparingly, explicit questions to group members. This may seem to go against the notion of direct observation, and more akin to interviewing ... but in participant observation you are less likely to have 'set piece' interviews and much more likely to have opportunistic 'on the wing' discussions with individuals.[294]

Observation is a tool that allows the researcher to describe, analyse and interpret that which has been observed. Powers and Goode (1986)[295] suggest that 'quality of life' is the product of relationships between people in particular settings. It is people's actions and behaviours that are examined and observation is all the more valuable when attempting a research study involving people with learning disabilities with a range of communication abilities. It is the directness of this methodology that is the major advantage; watching what people do and listening to what they say. Such directness both contrasts to and complements semi-structured interviews, not least because interviews are notorious for discrepancies between what people say they will do and what they actually do.[296]

Reactivity provides a way of observing the reactions of the group so as to learn about them: how they see the world and the social systems they have established within which they act and interact. Taking notes was an excellent way for recording what was *not* being said, the *non-verbal social interaction* taking place within a group, and as much detail as possible was recorded. The information that came from the interviews and observations was written up as descriptive observation; for example, describing the setting, the people, the events, the reason for the discussion and so on. Spradley (1980) suggests nine dimensions for collecting and recording descriptive data:

- space   layout of physical setting; rooms, outdoor spaces, etc.
- actors   the name and relevant details of the people involved
- activities   the various activities of the actors
- objects   physical elements: furniture, etc.
- acts   specific individual actors
- events   particular occurrence, e.g. meetings
- time   the sequence of events
- goals   what the actors are attempting to accomplish
- feelings   emotions in particular context.[297]

Acknowledging from the beginning what can contribute to a distortion or the possible biases that may arise, helps to counteract them. Lofland and Lofland (1984) suggest five main aids to recording materials which are:

(1) running descriptions: specific, concrete, description of events, who is involved, conversations, keep out any references (e.g. A was trying to get to B);
(2) recall of forgotten material: things that come back to you later;

(3) interpretive ideas: notes offering an analysis of the situation. You need notes addressing the research question, and ones which will add supportive or elaborate material;
(4) personal impressions and feelings: your subjective reactions;
(5) reminder to look for additional information: e.g. to check A and B, take a look at C, etc.[298]

Observational techniques are particularly useful for the present study, because they are ways in which the researcher becomes part of, and participates in, the activities of the service users adopting a position which in other circumstances would not be possible. Participant observation is a method of gaining contact that cannot be gained simply by using interviews. The following illustrates the valuable insight that participation observation can offer:

> . . . a researcher must first gain access to a group in order to be a participant observer. This was done by anthropologist Sue Estroff in an effort to learn more about the daily lives and problems of ex-mental patients, experiencing the drudgery and degradation of their daily routine. She worked at low-paid jobs (such as slipping rings onto drapery rods) that were the lot of these ex-patients. She took the powerful antipsychotic drugs that were routinely administered to them and had distinctive side effects such as hand tremors and jiggling legs. And she experienced the extreme depression and despair that result when one suddenly stops taking these potent drugs. From her position as participant in the subculture of these mental patients, she could observe the con games that characterised the relationship between patients and mental health professionals.[299]

By combining different approaches for the sake of understanding the group, the study becomes essentially ethnomethodological in nature, linking interviews with asking questions and listening while observing.

This chapter seeks to explore the nature of the relationships between users, parents and carers and the professionals through an analysis based on observation.[300] To achieve this three different types of learning disability meetings in the council were selected because of their contrasting mix of users, parents and carers, professionals and committee members, also the formal and informal approaches they offered:

(1) The first choice was the main day centre in the borough: a modern, large and well-equipped building that can accommodate 50 users, plus staff. The meetings at the day centre aimed to be service user-led with the staff acting as facilitators.
(2) The second forum chosen was the learning disability liaison group. This brought together users, their families, carers and the professionals. These meetings were designed as a platform for the professionals to let

everyone know what proposals were being put forward for current and future services. The idea was to engage users and their carers thus enabling them to work equally with managers.[301]

(3) The third and final venue chosen was the social services committee held at the Town Hall. This was a formal meeting led by members of the council representing all political parties, who questioned senior managers about what was happening with services. Generally, these meetings discussed a range of issues concerning all council services, but on this occasion, and due largely to the negative press coverage, most of the meeting was handed over to the problems with learning disabilities services.

Observation sessions proved to be especially fruitful, because this was a turbulent time in the council's history of providing services to people with learning disabilities. Relations were particularly tense between council members, managers, users and their carers due to the publication in the local press of highly emotive articles critical of the lack of user consultation by social services management.

Recording observation sessions

For the majority of meetings at the day centre and the liaison group, the researcher sat at the back of the room and, with one or two exceptions, was introduced at the beginning of the session to the group, and the role and purpose for attending was made clear. It was explained that the interviewer was interested in the interaction at the meeting as well as the content. The opportunity for a question-and-answer session to talk about the research with staff and users and carers was offered before the meeting which, in many cases, developed into an informal conversation generally about the rights of people with learning disabilities. The information recorded included:

- the way communication operated between users and professionals;
- service users' behaviour towards each other and the way in which they addressed staff;
- the way staff engaged with the users and methods they utilised to encourage users to voice their opinions;
- the time users were given to respond and the way in which they were enabled to articulate responses (particularly interesting were the methods used to help people with sensory impairment).

Recording was carried out via a series of notations with three main themes which were: *Choice, Communication* and *Relationships with the Professionals.* Within each theme the results found variations of experience and individual accounts illustrate this. For example, carers seemed to experience wide variations in the support they received from virtually none to levels which were almost satisfactory. Other areas investigated were questions concerned with the reality of care plans in the context of budget constraints.

The day centre

Friday afternoon at the centre was a time of relaxation. Few formal classes were held and service users were free to meet with their keyworkers to talk through their timetable and other activities. Once a month staff organised a user group meeting where the main business was a general discussion concerning how users felt about their classes, and it provided an opportunity for people to suggest any changes they wanted to see happen. The discussion often included other aspects of people's lives outside the centre such as home life, respite care and transport. Two meetings at the day centre were attended with the second taking place two months after the first.

The first visit

The first meeting was held in the dining-room, because it was the largest space capable of accommodating all the users and staff who wished to take part on that day. There were 43 service users who attended and four members of staff: the manager and three keyworkers. The manager chaired the meeting and set the main agenda, but invited the service users to add any other items they wished. On this occasion no user did so. The agenda included:

(1) The taped newsletter that users made every month: the last newsletter was going to be listened to, so that ideas could be generated for the next news tape, due to begin later that week.
(2) The review of the day centre that had been carried out by managers and council inspectors was going to be discussed.
(3) The recent death of a service user and the funeral arrangements were to be talked about.
(4) Lastly, staff had been concerned about reports from users of bullying and a book had been bought on the subject by the manager: this was the final topic.

The discussion opened with the last item on the agenda. Users began straightaway to ask questions about bullying and expressed interest in the book. The manager said she had the book in her office, and people were welcome to go to the office and read it. She spoke about bullying saying: 'It is what we do to each other, and it is aggressive behaviour that can change over time as the bullying gets worse.' At the time this meeting took place, there had been a high-profile case in the media about a black female teacher who was being harassed and bullied by some of her pupils because of her ethnicity. The manager spoke about this giving it as an illustration of bullying and saying: 'Any users here who feel someone is bullying them must come and tell the staff straightaway so we can help and support you.' No user spoke about being bullied and it seemed the manager had included this item because it was a current topic in the news. The meeting then turned attention to item two of the agenda: the review of the day centre.

The manager said a review had been carried out by senior managers in the learning disability department along with social service in-house inspectors. She said what had come out of this review, when people were asked about the centre, was the fact they wanted a greater range and more choices of activities. The manager said: 'We are going to help you get more out of the centre beginning today by looking at the summer timetable.' The room erupted into loud laughter and clapping as the users showed their approval. The manager continued: 'You can help me by letting staff know your choices about what type of activities you want the summer timetable to include.' Almost immediately people began shouting out what they wanted to do. One person said: 'I like walking going down the road to the shops in the summer because it is warm.' The manager made some interesting suggestions herself for the timetable such as mountain climbing and deep sea diving. However, nobody showed much interest to these proposals. A keyworker suggested trips out to the park, or to the London Eye. Others put forward by another keyworker ranged from picnics to yoga. The manager asked the group which activities they would be most interested in doing by a show of hands, and proceeded to call out each activity in turn, as hands were raised and lowered. She explained that discussions about improving the range of summer activities at the centre would be taken up at the next staff meeting so that staff could also make comments. Users would be told what improvements staff thought could be made.

The manager then changed the subject and moved on to the next agenda item saying: 'Something sad has happened since we had our last meeting, something sad that made us cry. Somebody who used to come here to the centre who had very profound disabilities has died.' A woman with communication difficulties began making what can only be described as a loud yawning noise, a long drawn-out 'aaaaaa . . . mmmm' sound. This had a disturbing effect on many individuals in the room. She was obviously distressed and was comforted by a keyworker. The manager said that the man had died suddenly in hospital. The room was quiet as everybody listened intently to what was being said. The member of staff who had been keyworker to this user was invited by the manager to talk about what would happen at the funeral. The keyworker spoke about what happens at a funeral, the coffin and flowers, and said: 'Although we won't be able to see him again, we can share our good memories about him with each other here at the centre.' A user called out from the back of the room: 'He always liked to help people.' To which the keyworker replied: 'Yes that's right he did, he was thoughtful like that.' The manager had written to the family on behalf of the staff and service users, and before posting it she read it out to the group for their approval. From time to time individuals remembered something about the dead man and would call out spontaneously memories they had: 'He did pottery', shouted a user.

The manager offered several suggestions about what could be done as a memorial in honour of his life. Planting a tree was received by the users with enthusiasm and they agreed to do this. It was noticeable during the meeting that for the most part, users tended to be passive recipients of the manager's proposals and suggestions.[302] Although the subject of this man's death was clearly traumatic for many, the meeting did have its lighter moments. One man wanted to know: 'What's going to happen to his locker? I've had my eye on that for a long time. It's a good locker that is.'

The manager then turned her attention to talk about training the staff had been on recently. She spoke about the Makaton course some staff had just completed to help them communicate with users who had communication difficulties. One user stood up and showed the group the Makaton sign for 'dead'.

From the back of the room a man called out saying he wanted to discuss the menu. He said there was something at lunch that he didn't like. It was pancakes and he asked the staff to let him know when this was on the menu again and 'I'll bring my sandwiches', he said. The manager said the menu was set six weeks in advance, so it was no problem to read it to anyone who wanted to know and that way people could make their own minds up whether to have lunch at the centre or to bring along sandwiches. The manager brought the meeting to a close by summarising the main points. She said they had run out of time for today and the newsletter tape could wait until next time.

The second visit

For the second meeting, the TV lounge in the day centre was used instead of the dining room. Staff said it was more comfortable, although at first sight it resembled an office more than someone's sitting-room, with various pieces of equipment such as hoists and wheelchairs lying around. The walls were covered in timetables telling which users did what activity. On this occasion, the meeting was attended by the manager, two male keyworkers and 19 users. As with the previous meeting, an agenda had been set which included:

(1) the summer timetable;
(2) daily living skills;
(3) the newsletter and advocacy;
(4) transport.

This time the manager did not chair the meeting, but the discussion was led jointly by her and the keyworkers. None of the meetings was intended to be formal, but in comparison to the previous one, this meeting was more relaxed and less formal. This was perhaps due to the fact that people were in a lounge on sofas, not in a dining-room with hard wooden chairs and tables.

A keyworker began by saying staff had discussed ideas for the summer timetable and then she spoke briefly about some of the ideas. She said the previous meeting related to this one, and pointed out that on the walls around the room were parts of the new summer timetable, and as many of the users' choices as was practical had been included. Most people looked at the walls, but interestingly there were one or two service users in wheelchairs who had limited communication ability and posture problems, which meant they could not keep their heads up long enough to have a proper look at the walls. These people stared at the floor for most of the meeting only occasionally flopping their heads back, like rag dolls', to glance at the walls, before almost immediately letting their heads fall forward again and gazing into their laps once more. The keyworker offered different suggestions for the new timetable such as going to see a play in the West End. One young woman began to tell the group in detail what her timetable already was. The keyworker responded by saying: 'Your timetable will be changing now.' She continued by highlighting other choices that had been made for new activities such as cake making, gardening and soft toy making. The last suggestion brought tremendous laughs, shouts and whistles from members of the group.

A second keyworker spoke about daily living skills such as how to use the telephone. He said there were different classes at the centre designed to help people improve their independent living skills, such as the shopping group. He also spoke about more leisure activities which users had said they wanted, and promised that a dance group would be started later in the summer. One male user got up, went over to the manager and attempted to dance with her. Quite abruptly she responded by saying: 'Would you like to sit down?' Steadily throughout the course of the meeting more users and staff had joined in until the room was quite full. It was a very warm day in mid-June, and by this time the non-verbal users in the wheelchairs were sound asleep.

A third keyworker brought up the topic of the taped newsletter which was an agenda item carried forward from the last meeting. She said an item about advocacy was going to be included in the newsletter, and asked if any of the group had an advocate? Only one person said she did, and the keyworker said it was important to talk about making decisions with the help of advocates. She said this was especially important in relation to matters to do with health, such as teeth, and she suggested an article for the newspaper tape which could be called 'Plain Facts'. The manager began to tell the group about advocates and what they do. At this point about half the service users left to attend a specially arranged art workshop, which unsettled the meeting. A babble began between the service users, and the manager who was still speaking called for quiet. She turned to the non-verbal users, who due to the noise were now awake, and asked them to let her know if they wanted help from an advocate by lifting their hand, or smiling if they preferred.

Transport and the lateness of the buses was briefly touched upon. The users complained about the fact that they couldn't get to 'work' (the day centre) on time because of this problem. One person said his friend was ill and could not use the bus because he was so ill. At this point it was 3.30 p.m. and people were eager to get home, consequently the manager brought the meeting to a close.

The Learning Disabilities Liaison Group

The social services department produced a glossy pamphlet called 'Making a Difference: The Learning Disabilities Liaison Group' in which they set out the aims for and value of having the liaison group. It stated:

> The learning disability liaison group meets four times a year, giving users and carers the opportunity to talk face-to-face with Councillors about services. The group is chaired by a Councillor. The Councillors and professionals involved in these groups are keen to get across that the liaison groups are valued as a way of establishing a user perspective across all council services, not just social services. The groups are useful for Councillors to hear from service users about their problems and complaints, because these in turn help Councillors when talking with senior managers and officers about users' needs. They also act to inform Councillors and staff about what is not working. The group provides a way for users and carers to have an input into the work of the learning disabilities section, and offers real opportunity to meet others, exchange ideas and talk about issues. The process of turning the ideas and needs of service users into policy, which drives forward new services, is long and drawn out. It is also difficult to understand the political process of decision making. This is where the liaison group helps service users and carers to understand the processes involved. The liaison group sets out below a summary of the key issues for action that users, their families, staff and Councillors will be examining over the coming months.

Influencing other services

- joint meetings with the liaison group and the Health Authority;
- joint meetings of the liaison group on transport and welfare benefits.

Influencing the decision-making process about social services

- more accountability, with action points being followed up by councillors and staff;
- progress reports from the professionals on the action points.

Making a difference to the lives of service users

- quicker responses by councillors to action points;
- councillors to visit people in their own homes;
- tape recorders for councillors so they can hear the views of service users unable to attend the meeting.

Two visits were made to the liaison group meetings which were held one month apart. This was unusual. Normally the group met quarterly throughout the year. However, the second meeting was called due to the reports in the press relating to the suggested privatisation of the residential home Westbourne Crescent and other community-based resources mentioned in subsequent articles.

The first visit

Both the first and second meetings were held in one of the borough's large day centres for older people. What was striking was how big, cold and uncomfortable the room was. Many of the chairs were those normally found in old people's homes, high-backed plastic chairs. Bulbs did not have shades on them and, considering it was approaching winter, the room was not well heated.[303] Interestingly, no one seemed to notice this including the councillor.

Just over 60 people in total attended this meeting made up of four councillors, four managers including social and health care professionals, a senior manager from the Chief Executive's Office, ten representatives from local voluntary organisations, one advocate and around 30 parents and carers. The remainder, around 12, were service users.

The councillor chairing the meeting began by going through the notes of the previous meeting which were agreed by the professionals, families and service users. She set out the agenda items for the meeting which were:

- feedback from the liaison group away day;
- transport and the Best Value review;
- health for all.

Following this opening a senior member from the learning disabilities department stood up and announced that within the next few months the completion of the joint health and social care teams, coming together under one structure and housed in the same building, would be complete. She assured everyone that the services they received would not change, but added what was going to change would be the way the professionals were managed. Next a planning officer spoke about the away day the group had taken a few weeks prior to this meeting. He held up one of a number of leaflets that had been produced as a result of what people had said during the course of the day. He said:

'We need to think about the events of that day and the topics we talked about in our groups, because a lot of changes are going to be taking place in the Council that will affect all of us and this learning disabilities liaison group. Another area we looked at during the away day was transport and the problems people were having when using in-house and public transport to get to and from the day centre and the clubs. Some people had been spending up to two hours on a bus getting to the centre and home, but because most of you use public transport, it will remain a problem.'

A parent responded:

'This is a serious problem because our children are missing out on their classes. We were told something was going to be done about this. What about the people in wheelchairs? People are having to put up with two hours in the morning and two hours in the evening on the buses.'

The officer assured parents that managers were dealing with it, but he failed to say how or to inform the group of any progress that had been made since the last discussion. The councillor said that transport was being reviewed as part of the overall Best Value review taking place in the council. The aim of the Best Value review was to ensure that transport would undergo a real change, moving to become more service-user-orientated. He said:

'We have been having transport meetings and the next one is due in two weeks. At that meeting we will be talking about transport in terms of market testing and Best Value, and looking at new and improved community transport for our service users.'

A parent called out saying:

'The day centre was geographically in the wrong place. It is in one of the most congested parts of central London.'

The councillor responded that the essence of Best Value was to address the needs of the users and it is about bringing back the service to the users.

Up to this point the meeting had been led by the professionals. It was noticeable that no people with learning disabilities had contributed to the discussion.

A tea break was called for 15 minutes when people mingled together and the second half of the evening meeting was given over to the topic 'Health for all'.

A clinician practitioner from the learning disabilities joint team spoke about the needs of people with learning disabilities in relation to their health such as how to see the GP and how to look after themselves, also how to use the local hospital when needed. She spoke about the new partnership team with health and social care professionals and the single point of entry to all services for the users, via care management, which meant that users could have access to social workers, keyworkers, clinicians, psychologists and nurses, all housed in the one building. A user said: 'I saw my dentist last week' and then began rocking and laughing. The tone of the evening up to this point had been so serious that this comment brought light relief to the room and many staff as well as parents began laughing. It was one of those comments that for no understandable reason cause hilarity. Once this had died down the clinician continued to talk about research that had been carried out to look at the health needs of people with learning disabilities by the local health authority. She said: 'We wanted to meet with as many service users as we could to find out what their health needs were, so that we can do our job well.'

It was then suggested by the clinician that the meeting divide into three groups, and each group could talk about their health needs. She offered three areas that the groups might like to talk about which were:

(1) primary care trusts;
(2) health education;
(3) links with hospitals.

She asked the groups to consider the following questions:

(1) What health care issues are important to you?
(2) Where do you want to receive health care?
(3) Who do you want to help you with your health?

Breaking into smaller groups appeared the most effective way to involve the service users, and can possibly be attributed, in part at least, to the fact that it is a method they were familiar with, which they used regularly at the day centre and were therefore comfortable with. After about twenty minutes the clinician said: 'Time is up' and asked people to return to their original seats. Each group had elected a spokesperson who reported on what had been discussed in the groups.

Group 1

An officer represented this group, who said the group had talked about their own experiences of health services, and the most important part of using these services was having accessible information which was easy to understand. This could include such things as drawings. The group felt it might be a good idea for people with learning disabilities to have a regular 'all over' health check, which could include things that might otherwise get overlooked, such as a balanced diet, emotional health, hearing and skin conditions. Everyone should receive the health checks they need from their doctor, but some health checks could also be done at day centres or at health centres by dentists and opticians.

Group 2

Two service users helped by a health worker were the representatives for this group. The main discussion had been concerned with what partnership working could achieve in terms of meeting user needs, and they also looked at complementary medicine. As with the previous group, they also said there was a real need for clear information to enable people to have an informed choice. One user in the group had expressed his concern that people with learning disabilities were not offered the same choice in terms of health services as everyone else, like checks for prostate or breast cancer. A solution proposed by this group was a one-stop shop, and perhaps the new partnership arrangements would help with this. The group examined varying locations for receiving healthcare, not just doctors' surgeries, and saw GP practices as an important source of information about health, saying it was important that receptionists were well informed and well trained about learning disability issues. This might also solve other related problems some people had with getting new prescriptions or making a convenient appointment time.

Group 3

The results of the discussions from Group 3 were presented by a user and an advocate. The group reported back that there were a number of specialists such as chiropodists and dentists who helped people with their health needs. There were other complementary health workers, like aromatherapists, who might also be able to help people with their health. It was important to have good information about what was available so that people could make an informed choice. In addition, group members said that better access to gyms and sports centres would be something that might improve people's health. Some individuals had attempted to use the services provided by the joint health and social care teams, but had had negative experiences. One man, for example, said: 'There are lots of staff around but they are always too busy to help me. I want more staff because they are all too busy all the time.'

The clinician thanked everybody for taking part and for bringing such vital concerns to their attention. She said 'a number of important points had been highlighted that would be taken away for the professionals to work on'. These were summarised:

(1) the request for GPs and receptionists to be better informed about the needs of people with learning disabilities;
(2) the suggestion that health checks by a dentist or an optician could be made at day services, as well as 'one-stop shops' such as health centres;
(3) that good health includes better access to physical activity and exercise for people with learning disabilities;
(4) that good health includes better access to dietary advice for people with learning disabilities and their carers; and
(5) that service users and carers wanted quicker access to healthcare information and advice from the joint learning disabilities teams.

She said health and social services staff would be working together on the suggestions that came from the groups, and added:

'What we may need to do is be more flexible in our approach, like going out to the day centres rather than people always having to come into the department to see us. It may be possible for some health professionals to visit once a week to give advice. We may be able to set up a consultation group to discuss with the local doctors the health needs of our users.'

The councillor acting as chair thanked everyone for coming to the liaison group meeting. As the meeting broke up and people began to put on their coats and chatted with each other, there was a positive feeling and people seemed genuinely pleased with the meeting. Shortly after this the local press published the articles about the privatisation of Westbourne Crescent and other possible threats to learning disability resources, such as dramatic changes to day centres, and the supported living schemes. The subsequent meeting had a very different atmosphere.

The second visit

Just over 70 people turned up to attend the meeting, including councillors, senior managers, an advocate, a mix of day centre and residential staff from the council, and representatives from voluntary organisations in the borough. The last group of staff were representative of all levels within their organisations. Also present were parents, carers and users.

As with the previous meeting this one was opened by the councillor acting as chair for the evening. She began by stating that officers of the council, managers and keyworkers were not allowed to speak for the users and
continued:

> 'Our normal agenda has been put to one side for this evening, and
> instead I want to concentrate on the reports many of you may have seen
> in the press. I know a lot of you are wondering what is happening and
> this evening presents an opportunity to share with you our plans. I
> want to talk about your concerns for the proposed privatisation of
> Westbourne Crescent the press have reported, and questions about
> budget savings which have also been floated in the papers.'

The atmosphere in the hall was extremely tense and there was a general
air of anger as parents, carers and users muttered to one another. A user
stood up and agreed with the chair saying she supported the speaker.
Another service user angrily shouted out: 'We don't like being called mentally handicapped, we're not stupid you know.' A keyworker from one of
the residential homes said:

> 'The service users here tonight and people in general who use the serv-
> ices won't understand the process of what's going on and, therefore, it
> isn't a fair consultation process.'

A senior manager asked to speak and responded by explaining:

> 'Yes it is difficult and we realise there are a lot of feelings involved.
> What we are going to do is have a feasibility study carried out to help
> us understand and achieve the best way forward, and if necessary
> time-scales can be extended.'

Looking around the room there was considerable lack of interest from
service users who were greeting each other. One person turning to another
said: 'How are you?' Others with communication difficulties were making
noises or shouting out from time to time. Parents and carers had fixed
expressions as they listened intently to the chair and the senior management.
It was clear they wanted straight answers.

A manager who worked in strategic planning for learning disabilities
services said they were trying to arrange meetings with users and their families to talk about the proposed changes: 'So far discussions have not taken
place, I know, and I apologise for that on behalf of the department.' A parent clearly angry at the whole thing asked what about the £84,000 that had
been lost because the professionals had overlooked the claim: 'Couldn't that
be used then?' She said: 'You're taking that money away from the handicapped to pay for the incompetence of your officers.' During these

exchanges people were still coming in to the meeting and users continued to call out to each other across the room almost unaware of the general discussion. One man called out 'Jimmy' over and over again. He was mostly ignored until it became too much for parents and staff sitting either side who tried to calm him down.

The councillor moved the meeting on to briefly discuss related agenda items. The Supporting People initiative was talked about, and a manager said the learning disabilities department was beginning to work more closely with housing because of this new programme that the government was introducing. Those who spoke throughout the meeting were mostly professionals and councillors. It was noticeable that no service user made a comment, nor were there any visible signs that they were either encouraged or supported to contribute their ideas or ask questions. Interesting contradictions could be found between the themes running through these meetings. For example, one item that was discussed explored at length how advocates could effectively be used to help users participate, yet here was an ideal opportunity with no visible attempt being made to enable users to be included.

An overhead projector had been set up and one of the planning officers began to speak about day services. The projector was used to illustrate points, showing how services were connected such as social services and housing, also education and leisure. The officer said there was a process taking place around the activities day centres could offer for the future and it was a process going on at the moment. He continued by telling the meeting that a report would be produced about the future use of day centres and managers would be telling people what the findings of the report were. He said: 'One of the areas being looked at is paid work for people who currently go to day centres; 93 per cent of users said they would rather have paid work.' A user shouted out: 'Good idea computer computer.' The advocate asked the planning officer about people who had profound physical and communication needs and who use day centres. 'There are many unable to work who want to continue attending their centre.' The officer referred back to the report saying: 'We are expecting to publish our findings about the future of day services in the borough very soon.' After this a tea break was called by the chair. The tea break was interesting in itself, because it was the only time during the evening, which lasted a little over two hours, when officers and managers actively mixed with users speaking and getting their views about what was going on. This was less so with the councillors who mixed, for the most part, among themselves and with managers.

After the break a service user, who had not been present during the first part of the meeting, stood up and spoke. With the aid of his keyworker this man read out a letter which addressed the concerns surrounding the proposed privatisation of the supported living schemes. The scheme housed people in ordinary houses in the borough. Normally no more than five people shared a house with 24-hour live-in staff employed by the council. The service user, once he had finished reading, said: 'I'm so stressed with this business that I'm going to go away from this area and never come back.' There was loud applause and laughter from many users around the room at this comment. The councillor said it was not the intention to cause distress either to those living at Westbourne Crescent or those who used other services. The advocate asked about the privatisation of the supported living schemes, but the councillor avoided answering the question directly and instead assured the meeting that no final decision had been arrived at, adding: 'It was necessary for everyone to see this, not as a decision the Council is taking but as part of the wider government agenda for change in local services.' Various parents and carers were visibly angry and upset by this statement and asked further questions about services to people with learning disabilities in the borough and privatisation. The debate was intense and drew emotional responses from parents and carers alike. The councillor said: 'Nothing can move forward on any of these issues until they had gone before the social services committee.' One mother said of privatisation: 'It's like sacking the mothers and fathers to some of the most vulnerable people in the borough who relied on these services.' A user followed this by saying: 'I don't want to see this happen.' Another parent said: 'What you're talking about here is Best Value isn't it. And we know that means going for the chequebook. It is just about the price isn't it? It's the same as getting a load of cowboy builders in to do a job, but the difference here is you're playing with people's lives.' A manager who had spoken earlier answered this point. She talked about the consultation process, and said it was taking longer than people realised, and meetings like this were part of informing and consulting. One mother said: 'Half the people we are talking about here tonight can't even speak for themselves. They will have to go along with whatever decision you lot make, won't they?' Another parent agreed adding: 'Even the letters you sent out to us are complicated. Why can't you use language that can be understood?'

SOCIAL SERVICES COMMITTEE

All committee meetings are held at the Town Hall, and this was the case with the social services committee included for observation in the present study. The main council chamber, which had some resemblance to the House of Commons debating chamber, was occupied by councillors, managers, health professionals and a Unison representative, as well as the advocate. The councillors from the three main political parties sat facing each other ready to speak into their microphones. Officers of the council also had the advantage of using this equipment, but not people upstairs in the public gallery. Some people with learning disabilities sat in the main chamber but at the back, and a considerable way from where the councillor and managers spoke. In the public gallery were most of the staff from

Westbourne Crescent along with a mix of parents, carers and users. Parents and carers had banners hanging from the public gallery with slogans about the cost of services and denouncing New Labour, Blair and Gordon Brown. Mockingly one banner read: *This Council is a leading flagship Labour Council.*

The meeting was begun by the chair who asked for an update from the officers regarding the planned move of Westbourne Crescent from the management of the local authority to a voluntary sector provider. A manager responded by giving a brief outline of the progress that had been made, following which the Unison representative was invited to speak. He argued that the running costs of Westbourne Crescent had not been based on the principles of Best Value, and suggested it was a cost-effective home run by the council, which provided excellent 24-hour care to three users at minimal cost. He argued that the present quality of care was very high and parents wanted this to continue. The Unison representative asked:

> 'What has happened to choice and the principles of ordinary life in this Council? The staff team at the home are dedicated professionals who strive for excellence and for the users to have maximum independence by creating new models of care. They are highly skilled, highly qualified people. Residents felt well cared for and secure. Their friends, parents and advocates did not want the disruption that would be caused to their care or sense of well-being with a change of service provider.'

He called on the councillors not to put costs before quality saying: 'I ask all members here tonight not to support the motion.'

Next the advocate spoke. He said that the proposal was causing the people who lived at Westbourne Crescent a great deal of stress, and at this point a woman with learning disabilities sitting opposite him began crying. He asked what evidence there was to support the case for privatisation?

The next to speak was the brother of a woman, Linda, who lived at the home. He stood up nervous and unsure of himself and said:

> 'I mean on the one hand I hear good reports about the people who look after our Linda, and most of the families here want to keep the staff. There are underlying assumptions. With the way things are now we can see users' independence increasing. My sister Linda, for instance, she loves to go shopping, but can't catch a bus. She needs someone with her all the time. Let's have a review, eh, before you go ahead?'

A senior manager spoke next and explained a feasibility study was underway, examining the new community support model that was being proposed. The new voluntary organisation who were being considered to take over the management of Westbourne Crescent were committed to supporting people with learning disabilities in their local community. As she was speaking the staff from Westbourne Crescent shook their heads and 'boos' could be heard coming from the public gallery. The manager continued to list some areas that the study would examine such as hours and costings, and said it would include the concerns of parents and carers. A member of the Conservative group asked for a review of the study to be brought back to Committee in six months' time. Another Conservative member asked about the rest of the supported living schemes, and a third asked if consideration had been given to individual care assessments in light of the changes being put to council members. The senior manager replied by saying that a mental health assessment had been carried out on all the service users who were living at Westbourne Crescent, and she said the study would take into account care plans. A member of the Liberal Democrats questioned the time-scales and reminded officers that considerable anxiety was being experienced both by residents of the home and by staff working there. He said: 'We must not forget staff will be worried about their jobs.' Another councillor said: 'Isn't it the case that most service users are out during the day so where is there a need for a permanent staff team at all?'

Although at this point the meeting had not ended, it had proved enough for the staff of Westbourne Crescent and many parents, carers and users. In a dignified manner they protested by getting up from their seats and making their way out of the chamber.

The final person to speak was the director of social services who addressed the committee, saying:

> 'The council is responding to the needs of the service users rather than traditional patterns of working by staff. Now is not the time to talk about services to people with learning disabilities in our borough in terms of Best Value, but in four years from now when we can measure the true worth of these changes.'

SUMMARY

The group forums demonstrated that people with learning disabilities, their families and carers are keen to have a 'voice'. When they were included in discussions they portrayed a sense of openness and honesty, despite the difficulties and constraints they faced. The groups, however, did little to empower users and carers to take centre-stage; rather the professionals could often be seen as acting like gatekeepers controlling many of these situations. Two things were noticeable: first, the ages of the carers, who tended to be older people; and second, the lack of ethnic diversity represented. Support is needed to offer users and carers the opportunity to take an active lead in the discussions and decisions being made at group forums, helping them to grow in confidence. One message that comes from this study is that users and their families must be empowered to take control, and begin to bring about the positive changes in their lives, and in the services they want to improve those lives.

NOTES

294 C. Robson, *Real World Research: a Resource for Social Scientists & Practitioner-Researchers* (Massachusetts, MA: Blackwell Publishers, 1993), p. 313.

295 J. Powers and D. Goode, 'Enhancing the Quality of Life of Persons with Disabilities through Incentives Management', unpublished manuscript (New York: Rose F. Kennedy Centre, Albert Einstein College of Medicine, 1986).

296 S. Oskamp, 'Methods of Studying Social Behaviour', in L. S. Wrightsman (ed.), *Social Psychology*, 2nd edn (Monterey, CA: Brooks/Cole 1977), p. 191. D. J. Hanson, 'Relationship between Methods and Judges in Attitude Behaviour Research', *Psychology* (1980) 17: 11–13, 126 and 191.

297 J. P. Spradley, *Participant Observation* (New York: Holt, Rinehart & Winston, 1980), p. 31.

298 J. Lofland and L. H. Lofland, *Analysing Social Settings: a Guide to Qualitative Observation and Analysis*, 2nd edn (Belmont, CA: Wadsworth, 1984), pp. 22, 203, 297, 376, 388.

299 R. D. Monette, J. T. Sullivan and R. C. Dejong, *Applied Social Research Tool for Human Services* (New York: CBS College Publishing, 1986), p. 191.

300 Robson, *Real World Research*, p. 192.

301 Terry Philpot and Linda Ward, *Values & Visions: Changing Ideas in Services for People with Learning Difficulties* (Oxford: Butterworth-Heinemann, 1995), p. 181.

302 J. Raymond (ed.), *Empowerment in Community Care* (London: Chapman & Hall, 1995), p. 3.

303 Spradley, *Participant Observation*, p. 31.

7 Conclusion

THE STUDY AND ITS LIMITATIONS

For more than two decades, British governments have been committed to ensuring the civil and social rights of people with learning disabilities in part by attempting to guarantee for them choice and control over the way they live their lives through participation in planning their services. Yet practical experience suggested that in some cases some local authority attempts to involve people with learning disabilities in service planning lacked reality, because of the failure to acknowledge the problems of communication that affected some of those involved.

The purpose of this book was to explore the role of communication in explaining the apparently chequered performance of local authorities in meeting their statutory requirements to involve users and carers in service planning. The work is illuminated by illustrations drawn directly from the experiences of this group, their families and carers and the professionals involved in their support. It is their comments and discussions that make up the main body of the text. Qualitative research investigates subjective experiences with the purpose of understanding people's views of their social situation.[304]

When drawing up this project, key issues that were raised included an historical and present-day examination about how people with learning disabilities have been and continue to be represented: how they are defined and 'classified' and the part they play in advocating their rights to equality, were all adopted as areas for investigation. The impetus for the way in which the framework developed came from the service users and carers. Adopting a flexible approach, which used both semi-structured interviews and observation 'seeking to be an unnoticed part of the wallpaper',[305] was thought to further help users and carers to contribute to the discussion. It enabled them to offer their views and ideas about the important issues and concerns for them, which in turn influenced the developing research framework. This allowed the study to be different in two significant ways. Carrying out the research using both group observation and individual interviews, permitted both a 'collective' approach, where views were developed through forums, as in the case of day centre and liaison groups, exchanging and debating ideas, and also, complementing this, more personalised one-to-one accounts of individual experiences. Moreover, observation sessions offered invaluable opportunities for developing an understanding of how, in practice, the council was developing processes for involving people with learning disabilities in planning, and at the same time to make some assessment of the contribution to that process of those people interviewed, who were able to communicate sufficiently to participate effectively in the interviews.

PEOPLE INVOLVED IN PARTICIPATION AND PLANNING

The method adopted was one that encouraged users, carers and professionals to determine what was important to them in considering the nature of the relationships between providers and beneficiaries, particularly in the context of the participation of users and carers in service planning. In this, the study both attempted to respond to injunctions from academics and members of the disability lobby to redress the power imbalance between interviewers and interviewees in the field of disability studies – regarded as likely to be particularly acute in the case of people with learning disabilities – and to anticipate the government White Paper, *Valuing People*, which sets guidance for service development for people with learning disabilities and for research in this area.

Interviews with professionals, carers and users indicated a high level of commitment to the ideal of participation in planning and service development. Professionals, while acknowledging some difficulties with communication in planning contexts, nevertheless saw the process as essentially unproblematic. For them, the resistance of users and carers to provision changes was as important an impediment to progress as possible communication difficulties. This in itself indicated that there were problems besides those of communication which disrupted the participatory process in planning.

The observational sessions demonstrated the inability of the professionals to respond positively to the expressed needs of users and carers because of the constraints of ideology and resource requirements. But they also demonstrated, in ways not evident from interview material, the assumption among professionals that for users, participation was to be equated with *presence* at planning and other consultative meetings. No attempt was made to engage those with little or no spoken communication. Those with some speech, but with little apparent ability to formulate it into a coherent or considered contribution, were allowed to repeat words, phrases, or simple noises as an accepted contribution to the proceedings, as an expression of presence, rather than a contribution to discussion. Many of those with severe learning disabilities in wheelchairs, who found it difficult to raise their heads to make eye contact or to regard flip charts, remained with their eyes downcast, only occasionally rolling their heads back to take in the meeting visually. No advocate represented their point of view.

Professionals were not alone in their failure to include those with fitful or no verbal communication. Even those engaged in research tended to focus on people with whom they could communicate. It was a situation that created 'stars', those few people with learning disabilities who became practised, often with the help of advocates, at putting the 'learning disabilities view'. Even the present research, despite considerable attempts to include the full range of people with learning disabilities, was forced to focus, at least in the initial stages, on the local 'stars'. The observation sessions were crucial in helping to restore the balance to some degree. Even so, while it was possible to determine the nature of their participation, it remained difficult to determine the attitude of the people concerned towards these sessions, and impossible to know *anything* of their views towards the issues under discussion.

The data collected and analysed have been classified into three groups: what the service users responses were; how the professionals responded; and what the parents and carers said. In many ways service users see professionals as powerful figures of authority, which adds to the already existing complications for attempting to explore user involvement in service planning at any level. Therefore, an attempt was made to explore the role and nature of the relationship between the users and the professionals, seeking to investigate *if* and *how* the professionals broke down barriers that helped users to be involved in decisions, which ultimately have a direct impact on the service they receive. However, while most of the people with learning disabilities involved in this study came into contact with front-line workers, such as keyworkers and social workers, none mentioned being involved with staff working in strategic planning, or spoke about being consulted by professionals in more senior management roles.

The nature of choice and free will, relationships, and communication, was explored in this study and the complexities of 'subjective' and 'objective' definitions and understandings were highlighted. Limitations on social responsibility have been examined, linked to the broader discourse about the way in which people with learning disabilities have been labelled, and excluded from full citizenship.[306] Some individuals interviewed saw labels such as 'mentally handicapped' or having a 'learning disability' as offensive, stigmatising and unhelpful. Many carers argued these labels were necessary and truthful and often went on to clarify why they thought this. For example, one explained:

> 'We've lived through years of the names changing, it doesn't really change anything else just the names change. Truth is they're all handicapped in the end.'

Many people with learning disabilities spoke about the impact that negative labels had, and this was a theme which recurred in the interviews. One example came from a woman, now in her forties, who talked about how she felt at being labelled and the effect it had on her life:

> 'When I went to school they used to call me names and things. They said I was retarded and handicapped and then I got learning difficulties when I left school. I thought I was different but that isn't right is it? Do you think it's right to call me all those names? I expect that's why I can't get my own flat and job now. Do you think that was right?'

Other individuals felt being stigmatised had prevented their contributing to the wider society in the way they had wanted to. There was a real sense of being trapped and excluded as well as dependent both on others and on the state. This was true of carers and users alike. Both groups talked about the terms used in conventional discussions about them and in some of the groups when the term 'mentally handicapped' was used, people greeted it with a great deal of anger and frustration. An example was during one of the observation sessions described above (p. 158) when a user called out: 'We don't like being called mentally handicapped, we're not stupid you know.' It was difficult for users and carers to find a way of overcoming language that conveyed negative imagery about them. Even from the period when this study began to be written the 'label' changed again from that of 'learning difficulties' to 'learning disabilities', reflecting a long-drawn-out informal shift given formal recognition with the publication of *Valuing People*.

The project uncovered the feelings that parents and carers had towards the professionals. Despite limited opportunities, most parents and carers had taken part in some type of discussion group about services and had very clear views about where professionals were 'getting it wrong'. One mother said: 'It's the way the staff want it. They always do what they want anyway.' One predominant feature that did emerge was the number of parents and carers who felt the rapid and continual turn-over of staff did not help. One parent explained:

> 'You get it over and over again, the whole bloody thing starts over and over again. That's why we give up. You think you're getting somewhere with that one and then she leaves. Lo and behold in comes another even more enthusiastic than the last ready to set the world to rights. Six months down the road she gets promoted or leaves. A lot are agency you know, and . . . it's depressing that's what it is. You just get nowhere with them in the end.'

The feeling for many parents and carers as to the reasons they were not included in the planning process lay within a social/professional/institutional structure, rather than the responsibility being at an individual level. Many people spoke about what they and others did to try to challenge these constraints in order to improve their situation. It was notable throughout the research that the inability of both users and carers to achieve any real improvement is a measure of the continuing strength and success of these constraints. On many occasions users as well as carers referred in a negative way to consultation groups as 'talking shops'. The parent of a 50-year-old woman said:

> 'You tell me what gets done eh, nothing, they're all talk these people, talking shops that's all they are. I don't take our Christine no more. I told her during the winter. "The evenings are drawing in now," I said and "That's enough we're not going no more, Christine," I said and we never did go no more.'

Many parents and carers who took part in this study had for many years campaigned for changes. They all drew attention to the problems and agreed that there were difficulties to overcome. The most significant factor arising when talking with carers was a sense of *not knowing enough* followed by *a lack of self-confidence and experience* to make their voice heard. A further barrier was the 'meaning' that lay behind becoming involved. Becoming involved meant different things to different people: for some it was about being represented on decision-making bodies; others believed that it was to do with holding professionals to account; while others saw it as taking direct action by setting up breakaway groups attached to voluntary organisations. There was also a feeling among carers that if they were making the effort to become involved and to organise, then councillors, politicians and the professionals should listen to what they had to say 'and meet us half-way'. Most families as well as some professionals thought local politicians had a crucial role to play in supporting user participation.

Over the past couple of years there has emerged a growing dissatisfaction with the approaches traditionally taken to researching and analysing issues related to the lives of people with learning disabilities. This has become all the more clear in light of *Valuing People* and, as part of the overall aims, the White Paper proposes funding a research project called 'People with Learning Disabilities: Services, Inclusion and Partnership'. The project is one of six being proposed seeking to generate knowledge about how to successfully implement the proposals in *Valuing People*. The importance the government has given to the research can be seen reflected in the estimated £2 million budget which has been set aside. The hope is this will prompt new and innovatory ways for researching learning disabilities issues. Academics and policy makers within the disability movement have called for changes to the traditional approaches taken to research.[307] 'People with Learning Disabilities: Services, Inclusion and Partnership' will investigate:

- service delivery in health and social care and its effectiveness to identify elements of good practice, implementation and sustainability;
- social inclusion, including access to good healthcare, and the factors which create disability barriers in people's lives;
- organisation development to show how staff performance in learning disability services can be supported to achieve better services. [308]

The present small-scale case study was undertaken in part to try to develop an approach to research in this area which would meet to some degree the criticisms of the disability lobby. It was to this end that emphasis was placed on:

- enabling people with learning disabilities and their carers to contribute to the development and shaping of the research agenda;
- using a combination of group observations and one-to-one interviews;
- inviting participants to contribute their own concerns during the interviews and group debates.

The process of engaging users and carers in identifying the major themes to be explored was an attempt to ensure that it was their concerns and priorities which were reflected in the research. Yet the problems encountered, particularly with regard to communication, demonstrate how difficult progress beyond this point is likely to be.

THE PLANNING AND INVOLVEMENT PROCESS

The research draws attention to the fact that a common agenda is shared by users and carers. Many participants wanted their voice to be heard and made it clear that they were willing to become more actively involved in campaigning for their rights, especially in light of the hope *Valuing People* held out for them. There was a real sense of commitment and wanting to make change happen. Ostensibly, *Valuing People* offers a 'new politics' for people with learning disabilities for the 21st century, and the White Paper promises a transformation, revitalisation and a positive change within the politics of learning disability.

When this work began in 1998, few well-known research studies had been published which explored the relationship between people with learning disabilities and their inclusion in strategic planning and service development. It was a new area where both the literature and research had progressed little. Indeed, constant referral to the same small body of literature and small body of ideas ultimately became frustrating while the researching was in practice in the field. The present study began in the early days of local authority strategic planning, when people with learning disabilities had virtually no representation on planning boards. Now, however, all local authorities are required to implement strategies for involving users in the processes of planning, such as partnership boards. The research indicates some of the methods local authorities are likely to be forced to utilise in pursuing participatory goals and demonstrates how difficult it will be to implement *Valuing People*.

THE DISCUSSION SCHEDULE

Some parts of the research schedule were more successful than others, some questions being easier for people with learning disabilities to understand, although a great deal of time and thought had gone into making questions flexible and open. Thought was given before the interviews as to how questions could be rephrased for individuals if they did not understand them initially, or were unsure of the meaning. Within this work are a number of abstract concepts that can be difficult to grasp, such as the notion of 'choice'. Many people with learning disabilities found abstract ideas difficult, not least because talking about choice is relatively new in the lives of some of them. This caused practical problems such as people needing time to think about what was being asked of them. One failing in hindsight was that no pictures or images that could have helped were used during the course of interviews, but again this was to do with time limits on the interviews themselves. Most interviews took place at the day centre, and it was staff who controlled the length of time of each interview which normally was no more than half an hour. Service users were interviewed between classes when they were free or during coffee or lunch breaks.

Not all the questions in the schedule could be asked. There were a number of reasons for this. In some cases users wanted to talk about other experiences, developed from previous questions which were important to them. With professionals some questions were seen as being either too intrusive or inappropriate.

RECOMMENDATIONS FOR FUTURE RESEARCH

A wide cross-section of individuals with experience of people with learning disabilities took part in the research, but how 'representative' or 'typical' were their views in contrast to people's experiences more generally is a question that remains. One criticism expected of this study is that the people with learning disabilities were not typical because many were already 'activists' and to some degree this is true. A few, especially in the case of some parents, carers and service users, had been active participants in advocacy movements and campaigning initiatives for many years. Others had been involved in less structured social groups, such as religious groups and organisations, but most had not. Individuals who normally were not involved were actively sought. Sympathetic staff also proved helpful here, but of course it would be naive to suggest there is such a thing as a 'typical' parent, carer, user or professional.

It has been important for this study to challenge the stereotypes. Participants in the research ranged, in the case of people with learning disabilities, from those whose communication was limited to others who were highly articulate and independent. Parents, carers and users came from very different backgrounds. The council under investigation is that of one of the wealthiest inner London boroughs, and participants ranged from those who were very comfortable materially, to those who lived in poverty on some of the worst run-down estates in the country. True representation of any minority or marginalised group can only be made when more people have their say ensuring the widest possible range of views, and this is what the study has in part successfully achieved.[309] The problems of achieving true representation of this group, in terms of communication difficulties, is best seen with the example at the day centre of the young woman in the wheelchair who could not communicate verbally but raised her head from time to time to look around the room before letting it flop back and looking into her lap again, with nobody taking much notice of her.

A commitment to include in the planning process all the groups that were interviewed or observed raised a number of implications including: the need for advocacy support for some people to take part; accessible meeting-places; interpretation, personal assistance, clear/understandable information, including pictures, videos, audio cassettes, braille, signers, and ethnic minority languages. What this study demonstrates is the need to change the approach to practice and policy development. It suggests that the agenda is not whether people share the same view, but that their *differences* are acknowledged and included in the process. The importance of involving people in the development of their own services and the services that users want and that are relevant to their lives, underlines the value of listening to what they have to say and sharing in their experiences. This process not only informed the research but also acted as a method for those taking part to develop their own theories, express their knowledge, ask their own questions, and come to their own conclusions.

While the limitations of this project are recognised the conclusion must be that observation, participation, and interviews were justified methodologies. The research schedule successfully reflected the main areas of concern for those taking part. Many of the practical problems were to do with time. With more time and resources, solutions to these problems could be discovered during the early stages of any future research. *Valuing People* holds out a great deal of promise for the future, and it is hoped that this study will inspire others to pursue similar themes and so add to a clearer understanding of the lives, choices and needs of people with learning disabilities. What the present project demonstrates is the difference between policy and practice, and the importance to understanding this difference of, on the one hand, *funding* and, on the other, *communication*. Apart from political pressure nothing much can be done about altering funding. Communication, however, is different. Yet comparing the interviews of users and carers with those of professionals it became clear that users and carers felt the process of participation in service planning to be unreal for reasons unconnected with communication difficulties. Policy development might be predetermined for ideological reasons by central government or the local authority. An example was the decision by central government to replace day activities with employment. Other policy choices were predetermined locally for reasons of financial constraints, an example being the proposed closure of homes like Westbourne Crescent. And it was these difficulties, rather than those associated with communication, which users and carers identified as making a mockery of choice in the planning process both at the macro and the individual level. Initially, most had participated in the process with interest and enthusiasm. But inability to acquire the services they regarded as being necessary for themselves, and failure at the macro level to respond to user and carer preferences in policy options, left most people disillusioned to the point where some preferred to abstain from participation. Caught between ideologically determined preferences and resource constraints within the department, professionals found their room for manoeuvre too narrow to respond to needs as carers and users reported them. On the whole, users were less likely than carers to actually pull out of the process altogether, if only because attendance at meetings represented some sort of social engagement in lives in which opportunities of this kind were not numerous.

Nevertheless, communication difficulties were apparent both in reports of meetings provided by professionals, carers and users, and also in those participatory planning meetings which were subject to formal observation. Although included from the outset as part of the research strategy, in practice observation came to be seen as essential not only to provide a dimension of evidence additional to that of the interviews, but also as a means of obtaining information for those people who were unable to communicate verbally. All users contacted were keen to be involved in the study, and every effort had been made to include those who found spoken language difficult or impossible. However, despite adopting some of the strategies advocated by social psychologists to aid communication, and many attempts at rephrasing simple questions, few of the interviews with those with little or no verbal communication were successful. Indeed, the exercise suggested that social psychologists who make substantial claims for the possibility of communication with such people seriously underestimate the problems involved for anyone without extensive knowledge of the individual concerned.

Any attempt to improve the capacity of professionals to engage with *all* users in the planning process will require substantial outlay of additional resources: first, to develop more effective communication systems and to train professionals in them; second, to train and employ a sufficient number of advocates to represent the views of those with communication difficulties to redress the power imbalance in their encounters with professionals; third, to ensure enough time in meetings is available to make effective communication possible for everyone. However, it is clear from the present study that for participation in planning to mean more than the incorporation of users and carers into policy developments as determined by central and local authorities, sufficient resources will have to be made available for choice to be a reality, untrammelled by the preferences of professionals and policy makers.

NOTES

304 S. J. Taylor and R. Bogdan, 'A Qualitative Approach to the Study of Community Adjustment', in R. H. Bruininiks, C. E. Meyers, B. B. Lakin and K. C. Lakin (eds) *Deinstitutionalisation and Community Adjustment of Mentally Retarded People*, monograph 4 (Washington, DC: AAMD, 1981).

305 Robson, Real World Research, p. 194.

306 P. Beresford and J. Campbell, 'Disabled People, Service Users, Users Involvement and Representation', *Disability and Society*, 9, no. 3 (1994): 315–25.

307 M. Oliver, *The Politics of Disablement*, pp. 8–9. J. Morris, *Pride Against Prejudice* (London: Women's Press, 1991), pp. 130–3.

308 Department of Health, *Valuing People*, p. 114.

309 B. Glaser and A. Strauss, *The Discovery of Grounded Theory: Strategies for Qualitative Research* (New York: Aldine, 1967).

APPENDIX

A: THE RESEARCH DESIGN AND QUALITATIVE METHODOLOGY

INTRODUCTION

The purpose of the study on which this book is based is to investigate how adults with learning disabilities are involved in service planning. Communication is explored in order to analyse what happens during consultation meetings and planning procedures, and to get users' opinions about it. Because of the problems encountered with verbal communication in many interviews, and the difficulties involved with communication, it was decided that evidence would be collected through semi-structured interviews and group observations. Seeing people in different settings deepens understanding. The intention was to focus on how users, parents and paid carers take part in and contribute their ideas towards the development of the services they want. The present study, based on semi-structured interviews and group observations, intended to explore how people react to the services from which they are assumed to benefit.

The aim of the research set out to expose the experiences of users and carers in order to see to what extent they participate in the decision-making processes of the council involved in this investigation. Enabling users and carers to lead the research, by expressing their concerns and contributing their ideas, was the first step to giving them 'voice' to challenge the system. What was hoped was that participating in the study would be a positive experience for the individuals, and the research methodology was chosen because it was felt to be consistent with this approach. Participatory and emancipatory methods place emphasis on equalising the relationship between the researcher and the participant.[310] This style is also consistent with both the participatory and individualised approaches towards the development of a qualitative design. The intention of using a qualitative design was to gain the views of individuals about the key objectives of policy within a flexible framework, and the mechanisms involved in exploring their own ideas around choice and social inclusion.

The methodology evolved through the interviews and observations, and highlighted the experiences of people using social services. The definitions of choice, communication and social inclusion are themes which the research sought to explore with those involved in the study. Rather than a prior definition being given to these terms throughout the research, people's own definitions emerged and were utilised. No claims are made that those who participated in the research are representative of all people with learning disabilities and their carers, but an attempt was made to involve as wide a selection of people as possible. The way questions were worded was tailored to the communication skills and cognitive abilities of each person.

The field study sought to examine if and how the council's social services department included users and carers in service planning, and to investigate the council's consultation mechanisms to see *how* the choices of users with learning disabilities were addressed. Apart from the question of communication itself, there were also problems relating to tensions inherent in a policy that requires both consultation and the expression of choice, but within a framework of severe resource constraints. How do professionals address the awkward situation where they are encouraging the setting-up of consultation meetings and publicising the consultation process, but at the same time trying to find financial savings which in one year alone totalled £200,000 for learning disabilities services in the department?

Five main groups of people were invited to participate in the study:

(1) individuals with learning disabilities who use the services;
(2) professionals working at various levels within the council's social services department;
(3) parents;
(4) paid carers;
(5) advocates.

The field study was directed at exploring the government's expectation on local authorities to develop user-led services. At the same time it was hoped to highlight contradictions between the government's expectations on local authorities to develop social services, and government financing of these services.

THE FIELD STUDY

Interviews

The interview format is important because it is known to affect the respondent's answers and there are certain responses during an interview to which people with learning disabilities are particularly susceptible. The tendency to want to please by responding affirmatively to a figure of authority, regardless of the context or question, is particularly prevalent in people with learning disabilities. The way a question is phrased, therefore, is of great importance. This highlights the need to be aware of the power imbalance between the individual with learning disabilities and the researcher.[311] Interviews are a social interaction and as far as possible, during the course of this study, they took the form of a relaxed social conversation. However, for some individuals even social conversation can provoke anxieties linked to:

- fear about meeting a stranger;
- uncertainty about the purpose of the interview;
- worry that the interviewer was from an institution that the user would be taken to following the interview.[312]

To combat any sense of anxiety the questions used simple and clear language, and the interviews were kept relatively short, taking on average half an hour. With other groups, such as the professionals, the interviews were considerably longer, usually taking around an hour.

Information given to the service user about the aims of the research was presented in a clear context in an attempt to further avoid producing high levels of anxiety or confusion. The participant had control over the questions she or he wished to answer, and if he or she wanted to end the interview. Encouraging people to develop their thoughts and ideas when they said something by responding with a 'yes' was important. Keeping eye contact and smiling helped to relax the person, putting them at ease, and further aided communication.

Semi-structured interviews were used with all participants and had a fluid agenda with open-ended questions allowing the respondent to give as much information as possible. This approach was especially important when interviewing people with learning disabilities, because of the problems concerned with their cognitive and communication abilities. The interview became an adaptable and flexible method for eliciting information. A strength of this form of interaction is language itself. Robson (1993) observes that: 'The human use of language is fascinating both as a behaviour in its own right, and for the virtually unique window that it opens on what lies behind.'[313] The cognitive ability of people with learning disabilities varies enormously and for this reason, the most appropriate methods combined semi-structured interviews and observation research.

The interviews with service users took place mainly in the council's largest day centre, because settings like this allowed service users to be interviewed in relaxed and familiar surroundings. Semi-structured interviews offered the further option of following up responses and investigating underlying motives in a way that other methodologies, such as observation, do not always provide. Questions were modified during the interviews depending on what seemed appropriate, and depending on which groups were being asked what questions. Robson (1993) offers four points to consider when carrying out semi-structured interviews:

- listen more than you speak;
- put questions in a straightforward, clear way;
- eliminate cues which lead interviewees to respond in a particular way;
- enjoy it;

and some questions to be avoided:

- long questions;
- multiple-barrelled questions, e.g. What do you feel about current pop music compared with five years ago?
- questions that involve jargon;
- leading questions;
- biased questions.[314]

Open-ended questions were particularly helpful when interviewing service users and Cohen and Manion (1989) outline the advantages of this approach:

> ... they are flexible; they allow the interviewer to probe so that he may go into more depth if he chooses, or clear up any misunderstandings; they enable the interviewer to test the limits of a respondent's knowledge; they encourage co-operation and rapport; and they allow the interviewer to make a truer assessment of what the respondent really believes. Open-ended situations can also result in unexpected or unanticipated answers, which may suggest hitherto unthought of relationships or hypotheses.[315]

Informed consent and confidentiality

Two main ethical concerns for social science research are *informed consent* and *confidentiality*. The first concern is about protecting the identity of those taking part in the study when the findings are made known. For this reason all the names used throughout this book are fictitious: this applies equally to people as well as place-names and organisations. Confidentiality was explained and made clear to everyone taking part at the beginning of the interviews, and they were told that their names would not be available to anyone else. It was essential that informed consent had been sought at the beginning of each interview, but this in itself presented problems. A crucial question that has been debated by academics, policy makers and advocates for years is: *How can people with learning disabilities give consent?* Critics have explored this question and the inherent difficulties associated with obtaining consent from people with cognitive and communication difficulties.[316]

For the purpose of this study, consent was sought by first of all asking the individual if he or she was happy to take part, and if so, did she or he want someone else present during the interview. Secondly, the people were, at various times throughout the interview, asked if they wished to continue, and if they were comfortable with the questions. Where communication was a problem the interview was terminated as soon as someone appeared to be uncomfortable. In a similar way parents and the paid carers were told that they could end the interview at any point they wished to do so, and at the end of each interview they were invited to make comments. Most said it was an enjoyable and thought-provoking experience.

The participants

There were 85 men and women with learning disabilities who participated in the study. They ranged from individuals described as having 'mild' learning disabilities and others with 'moderate' learning disabilities to a small proportion who were classed as having 'profound' learning disabilities that included varying degrees of speech, communication and cognitive impairment. Their ages ranged between 24 and 83. The service users who participated came from the researcher's contact with team managers in the learning disability section, the day centre manager, and carers in the adult placement scheme. A cross-section of participants was sought, and it was also important to include users and professionals who could represent the different stages of involvement in the planning and consultation process.

In the study 43 professionals, working at different levels throughout the hierarchy of the combined health and social care department, were interviewed. They included: joint commissioning managers, service managers, team leaders, care managers, brokers, the manager of the day centre, adult placement officers and keyworkers. From the health section came: a clinical psychologist, an occupational therapist and a speech and language therapist.

The total number of paid carers interviewed was 15, while 12 parents also agreed to be interviewed. Finally, one advocate was interviewed who was responsible for a large advocacy organisation jointly funded by two central London boroughs. In all a total of 156 people were interviewed.

Interviewing the service users

Interviews with service users were conducted at the main day centre in the borough. The day centre manager often determined when and where the interviews took place. Other venues included an evening social club and a summer social scheme. These last two venues were run by the voluntary organisation Octa, but financed by the local authority.

Service users included in the study were contacted through the day centre which accommodates around 50 users plus staff, and through the clubs. These clubs catered for up to 30 people with learning disabilities and often a significant number of parents also attended. At each establishment staff were in a position to know which service users would be interested in taking part, and if having an advocate present would be helpful. However, it was essential to establish from the beginning the role of the advocate and acknowledge the effect of having a third person present at the interview. During each interview the user's responses were written down verbatim by the researcher which was important because it allowed for the inclusion of communication and expression in the form of gestures and facial expressions to be recorded, which cannot be captured by other methods such as the use of audiotape. With any research expectations inevitably colour the researcher's view and have the potential to affect the interpretations of the situation, therefore starting with and maintaining an open mind was essential. Using simple, direct and open questions ensured clarity for the respondent. If, after a time, no response was forthcoming or the individual appeared confused or nervous, the question was reworded.

The researcher was invited to attend the day centre by the manager for two hours on a Friday afternoon when there was less activity in the way of classes taking place. This allowed some flexibility with staff and users but none the less was restrictive in the sense of the time allowed. Building trust and a rapport with the respondent was an essential part of the exercise and taking time to do this was important. This helped the researcher to gain some understanding about the individual, and an insight into his or her responses. It further allowed the development of a relaxed two-way conversation to take place.

Interviewing the professionals

The professionals were interviewed at their place of work. Commissioning managers, care managers, and health professionals were all office-based. Team leaders and keyworkers were interviewed at the day centre. With all groups the aims of the study were explained, along with other related issues such as ethics and confidentiality. On a number of occasions it was surprising just how open and honest the professionals were willing to be when they responded to questions. For example, one senior manager, when asked about involving users in decisions about service development, replied: 'Well if they can't contribute to the consultation and it's just a nice day out for them that's fine.' What was interesting about this statement was the fact that the manager did not talk, during the course of the interview, about any attempt to actively seek ways to involve service users.

The mix of professionals allowed for the emergence of greater variations between the responses made by keyworkers, as people working on the 'front line', and, in contrast, the responses given by senior office-based managers. Again the formats used with the professionals were observation sessions combined with semi-structured interviews which enabled participants to explore the key themes of the research: how people with learning disabilities are included in the decision-making process when planning services; the problems experienced with communication; and the relationship between service planning, choices and budgets.

The themes under investigation differed depending on the professional being interviewed. Keyworkers, for instance, were asked about a typical year with their users: holidays, birthdays, shopping, money, pubs, Christmas and so on. What was sought at this level was to find out *if* and *how* keyworkers facilitate inclusion in the normal rhythms of the year, enabling everyday choices to be made, examining the *normal patterns of life* discussed in the Jay Report (1979). Respecting the rights of the individuals using the service while also meeting their needs was being examined here.[317] How did these workers approach the idea of normalisation and go about making a month typical or a year normal for their user? Do service users have control over everyday aspects of their lives from a choice of the meal they want to how they handle their own money? How, if at all, did keyworkers support people with profound/multiple communication disabilities to make choices?

Again the day centre and clubs were used to interview keyworkers and conduct group observations. The reason for this combination was that day centres tend to set up structured discussion forums with set topics, and a timetable to be explored. The purpose of these meetings is usually to talk through ways users can develop a better understanding of what it means to be more independent. In contrast the evening club was centred around leisure and relaxation. In this way the field study explored two different perspectives of everyday life for people with learning disabilities.

Interviewing the parents

The government's commitment to increasing help and support to families and carers in recent years, is most clearly demonstrated through the publication of four major pieces of legislation. The first was the NHS & Community Care Act (1990); the second, the Carers (Recognition and Services) Act (1995).[318] Thirdly there was the publication of *Modernising Social Services, Promoting Independence, Improving Protection, Raising Standards* (1998),[319] and finally *Valuing People: A New Strategy for Learning Disability Services for the 21st Century* (2001).

The NHS & Community Care Act (1990) was the first piece of legislation that recognised the role of the carer, and the second was the Carers (Recognition and Services) Act (1995) which sought to redress previous imbalances by giving carers the right to an assessment and placing responsibility on local authorities to take into account the results of that assessment. It was expected that this approach would be more holistic because it recognised the needs of both the *carer* and the *user* separately. It further sought to build upon existing community care legislation, aiming at a shift in practice by placing a duty on local authorities to listen to the views of the carers, taking into account the ability of carers to provide and continue to provide care.[320] The Act covered three types of carers: adults caring for other adults, parents of sick or disabled children and young carers (aged under 18).

The White Paper *Modernising Social Services* (1998)[321] acknowledged that it had often been the case that services were not planned in a way that would ensure carers and users benefited most. The Act recognised that carers have separate needs saying their needs are often as wide-ranging as those of the people they are caring for. It praised the work of carers as being valuable, saying this has often gone unnoticed in the past. In 1998, the Prime Minster announced the development of a National Carers Strategy, with the aim of taking comprehensive views of activities in support of carers. An integrated strategy of action by the government was set out with the following key objectives:

- to empower carers so that they have more say about the types of services that they and the person they care for need;
- to consider how carers who work can be best supported so that they can remain in employment;
- to consider how the health needs of carers can better be met by the NHS and especially primary care groups;
- to see how communities can better support carers especially through volunteering.[322]

The government's most recent pledge to support carers of people with learning disabilities is outlined in *Valuing People* and seeks to 'increase the help and support carers receive from all agencies in order to fulfil their family and caring roles effectively'.[323] As with previous government publications the White Paper acknowledges the lifelong commitment that caring for a family member with learning disabilities means and a commitment without which the person with learning disabilities could not often continue to live in the community. *Valuing People* estimates as many as 60 per cent of adults with learning disabilities live with a family member, of which an estimated third of carers are aged 70 or over. The government sees its responsibility towards carers as enabling them to:

- receive the right support to help them in their caring role;
- obtain relevant information about services;
- know who to approach for advice and help;
- make their voices heard at national and local level.

The White Paper underlines the importance of training carers, and believes this is an invaluable two-way process whereby professionals can learn from the first-hand experiences of carers.

In light of these policy strategies similar themes were investigated, during the course of this study with carers and families. Semi-structured interviews were used with carers in their own homes coupled with observation techniques carried out at the learning disability liaison group meeting, as well as the social services committee meeting at the town hall, where council officials and members discussed the future direction for learning disability services in the council. The research examined the experiences of parents and carers when it came to being included in strategic planning. The interviews were adapted in a way that made them suitable for this group of participants.

Interviewing the carers

Most carers who were interviewed belonged to the Adult Placement Service which offered long-term, respite and day placements. The Adult Placement Service placed users in the homes of paid carers, who received a weekly 'fee' on a scale of between £200 and £400. Strict criteria determined the rate at which the carers were paid: for instance, to qualify for the higher rate, service users generally would have to demonstrate seriously challenging behaviour. In one case the user regularly smashed all the furniture in her bedroom. There were further conditions on the amount paid. From the weekly 'fee' the carers had to pay for extra overheads incurred while the individual was staying with them such as lighting, heating and laundry. The carers were required to buy food and toiletries for the user, and also carers had to arrange for the payment of their own tax and national insurance contributions. Many carers complained that employing an accountant once a year to carry out this was very costly. The service also arranged for carers to go into the homes of service users who live independently, and teach them to cook, shop and self-care. The questions asked of these carers explored the degree to which they were listened to by professionals and the support they received from the statutory sector: their experience of being included in service planning discussions and whether they felt that the overall process had any long-term effect for changing the types and quality of service delivery.

Interviewing the advocate

One advocate was interviewed but this person had responsibility for managing a large organisation that spanned two central London boroughs. This was a well-resourced and impressively run organisation. The advocate was interviewed in his office.

RESEARCH ETHICS

As with many research projects ethics were of central concern.[324] This was a particularly sensitive issue when involving individuals with communication and cognitive difficulties. In many cases topics that participants chose to talk about were of a highly personal and sensitive nature to them, and it was important that the names and other details of individuals who took part were changed or that they remained anonymous. There were other related ethical issues that had to be addressed: because of using observation and interview techniques, the 'rights' of the participants needed to be kept at the fore and were paramount, especially their right to have their views and feelings reflected as accurately as possible, uninfluenced by the judgement of others. A lack of time and resources prevented any attempt to structure the sample in such a way so as to reflect particular experiences arising from gender, class or ethnicity. With all the groups there was a difficulty about the nature of their relationship to each other; for example, parents, carers and people with learning disabilities often appeared reluctant to criticise the professionals. One participant talks in positive terms about the support she received, but there was an underlying sense of dissatisfaction:

'My dealings with social services have only been for a couple of years, but I found each section to be competent and willing to help. The first professional I dealt with was my support officer. His vast experience was invaluable. He always dealt with any problem with a professional stance. When he could not help he knew the various sectors in the department that could. Also letting me know the results beforehand of any events that relate to me as a carer, and generally keeps in touch. One flaw, certain sections of staff changes occur too frequently. This I hope in future will improve. The social worker and me didn't click at the beginning, but the broker was good to talk to. But no, the social worker wasn't that good really.'

NOTES

310 M. Oliver, *Understanding Disability: From Theory to Practice* (London: Macmillan, 1996).

311 M. Rosen, L. Floor and L. Zisfein, 'Investigating the Phenomenon of Acquiescence in the Mentally Handicapped', *Journal of Subnormality* 20 (1974): 58–68.

312 L. M. Grey and J. Jenkins, 'Investigating Service Satisfaction among People with Learning Difficulties', *Clinical Psychology Forum* 67 (1994): 20–2.

313 Robson, *Real World Research*.

314 Ibid., p. 232.

315 L. Cohen and L. Manion, *Research Methods in Education*, 3rd edn (London: Routledge, 1989), pp. 229, 233, 241, 439.

316 C. D. Morris, J. N. Niederbuhl, and M. Mahr, 'Determining the Capability of Individuals with Mental Retardation to give Informed Consent', *American Journal on Mental Retardation* 98, no. 2 (1993): 263–72.

317 Jay Report, *Committee of Inquiry into Mental Handicap Nursing & Care*, Vol. 1. Cmnd 7468-1 (London: HMSO, 1979).

318 Department of Health, *The Carers (Recognition and Services) Act.* (London: HMSO, 1995).

319 Department of Health, *Modernising Social Services, Promoting Independence, Improving Protection, Raising Standards.*
320 Carers' National Association, *'Still Battling?': The Carer's Act One Year On* (London: CNA, 1997), p. 9.
321 Department of Health, *Modernising Social Services*, p. 9.
322 The terms of reference for the National Carers Strategy are: to draw together existing work within the government that impacts on carers; to take account of the emerging findings of the Royal Commission on long-term care; to gather examples of best practice in providing help for carers at local level; to assess whether any key needs of carers have been overlooked; to clarify the government's objectives for carers; to set out an integrated strategy for future action by government; and to report through the parliamentary Under-secretary of State for Health to the Prime Minister.
323 Department of Health, *Valuing People,* p. 53.
324 Martin Bulmer, *Social Research Ethics* (London: Macmillan, 1982). H. Dean (ed.), *Ethics and Social Research* (Luton: University of Luton Press and Social Policy Association, 1996).

APPENDIX

B: THE SEMI-STRUCTURED DISCUSSION SCHEDULE

As previously discussed, the widest range of professionals was sought from across the spectrum of learning disability services and included: the head of the Learning Disability section along with the senior management team. Team managers for the social and clinical teams were interviewed, and within the clinical team also came a psychologist and a speech therapist. Other professionals, who agreed to take part in the research, were strategic commissioners, contract managers and two members of the brokerage team. Participants from front-line services included keyworkers and support workers, and also staff working at the day centre. One advocate was interviewed from an independent advocacy agency, but it is important to point out that the funding for the organisation and his post came directly from the local authority. The content of interviews varied according to the role and responsibility of the person being interviewed. The overall content of each interview varied depending on the particular topic; however, the core questions for each category all related to the key themes under investigation.

INTRODUCTION

The researcher introduced himself at the beginning of each interview with professionals, parents and carers and they were given a card on which was written an explanation about the aims of the research. At this point in time the study was called '"Listen to Me!" Involving People with Learning Disabilities in Service Planning & Development'. Once the participant had read the information she or he was invited to discuss it further if they wished. Most chose to focus on the questions included within the semi-structured interviews. The card they were given to read said:

> Policies for people with learning difficulties have emphasised the importance of their involvement in the planning of their own services. The aim of this study is to explore some problems that arise when attempting to include users in service planning. This research is interested in listening

to what people have to say who have first-hand experience of planning and using social services in this borough. This research is essentially about *communication* and *choice* between service users and professionals, and communication between workers and parents/carers. What is being examined is the council's planning procedures, so as to find out how services are developed as a direct response to the choices and wishes expressed by users. The research investigates this in light of Central Government policy especially the influence *Best Value* has had on service planning and the White Paper: *Valuing People*. What you say will be written down verbatim and at the end of this session it will be read back to you to make sure it has been recorded accurately. There isn't a questionnaire because hopefully we can turn this interview into a two-way conversation based on the main topics of choice, communication and social inclusion. Of course you have the final say on how the discussion develops and what you want kept out of the study. The research is completely confidential and no names will be used during any part of the study or subsequent publication(s). Thank you for agreeing to take part in this research.

SCHEDULE QUESTIONS

(1) Professionals

How do you involve people with learning difficulties in decisions about their services?

What do you see as their main expectations around service planning?

How do you go about ensuring the views of your users are (a) elicited and (b) understood?

What do you see as the key problems in the situation where a user expresses a choice about wanting a service that you know you cannot meet because of cost?

What role do families, carers and advocates have in the consultation process? What relationship do you have with family members and carers?

There were variations on the questions put to some professionals for the purpose of allowing greater clarity, and it was important to keep these questions quite straightforward and simple. For example, there were specific questions which focused on aspects of service provision associated with particular professionals:

What is brokerage?
What relationship does brokerage have with service users?

RESPONSE: Basically we are responsible for negotiating contracts and costs for the care manager, residential services, respite that sort of thing. One of the ideas is for costs to decrease as the user becomes more independent . . . There is no relationship with them, because that's the job of the care manager, OTs and other people who work closely with them.

What future direction do you think brokerage may take, and how do you see its future in light of developments such as direct payments to service users and the introduction of commissioning and contract services?

RESPONSE: The future is bright for brokerage. I feel the use of brokerage is going to increase as more is privatised and externalised.

Questions to keyworkers and support staff were also modified. Here are two examples:

Can you tell me a bit about a typical year for the person you support: events such as holidays, birthdays, Christmas and so forth. The normal rhythms of the year? How do you help your service user regarding choice and involvement in everyday activities?

What problems do you face when it comes to everyday choices with people who have little or no speech?

(2) Parents and carers

With parents and carers the questions asked sought to gain an overview of the life of the person with learning disabilities, and the relationship the family member had with professionals. The following are examples:

You said he has challenging behaviour?

RESPONSE: Yes that's right he does. When he gets distressed he will. . . .

And what about the staff?

RESPONSE: There is a rapid turnover and a lot of individual attention is difficult. . . .

You have spoken a little about the professionals you come into contact with, would you like to say more about other experiences you have had with them?

RESPONSE: Oh years ago it used to be really good. The communication between carers and service users with professionals has diminished over the last ten years.

(3) Service users

Interviewing service users was as expected the most difficult, and for this reason the questions were as open as possible. Some examples of this have already been given in the body of the study (see Chapter 3). It was important that questions were not put in such a way that a 'yes' or 'no' answer was an option in terms of a response, but that the questions automatically engaged the person in a two-way conversation. Here are some examples:

So who helps you get what you want or need?

What about a social worker helping you to make choices about things you want?

You said you wanted help getting a job – tell me a little bit more about that?

RESPONSE: 'Lynda she helps me get a job. Do you know Lynda? She's getting me a job cause I'm intelligent you see.'

Bianca, you said you very much enjoy working with older people. Can you say a little about how you got this job?

RESPONSE: 'Call me B for short. I work for the council: I'm a laundry assistant for the elderly. I've been there nearly 15 years. I started 24 November 1986. We've got the next liaison group meeting here at the home, did you know that?'

Difficulties encountered during the interviews with service users

In summary, it is important to highlight that attempts were made to include a cross-section of users including those people with communication difficulties. However, some had such profound communication difficulties that they either did not understand what was being asked of them or could not respond in a manner that could be understood by the interviewer. Others had a short attention span which made the interview process time-consuming and often resulted in the interviews having to be abandoned. Here are five examples of the type of communication and cognitive problems encountered.

Example 1: Thembia

'Yeah like the summer scheme. What's the time man? Coffee break coffee break? What's time man? What time? Do puzzles? I know the seaside. [*Uses very strong language.*] I like swearing man I like it. What's the time man what time? What we do this afternoon what we do? Er. No swearing eh? [*Again uses strong language.*] What time we make coffee? Man what day tomorrow? Are you going for a walk this afternoon man? Yeah to the park. Can we put the cooking on this afternoon man? What time the Wimpey man what time. [*The question was repeated seven times in a row.*] Did you go to the toilet? [*Swears.*] What's the time man?'

Example 2: Geraldine

- *Do you like it here at the day centre?*
- Here.
- *Do you like coming to the centre?*
- Here.
- *What do you like best?*
- Here. [Sings]. water, water, water.

Example 3: Samantha

- *What have you being doing today?*
- Been to work.
- *Do you like working?*
- Yea.
- *What are the staff like?*
- The staff – £3.00.
- *Is that your wages?*
- Sticking labels.
- *Do you have a keyworker?*
- Yes Dorothy.
- *What did Dorothy say?*
- I'm a star.

Example 4: Bob

- *Do you live with anyone?*
- White door 108. I live with mom on holiday Ireland aeroplane.
- *Who are you staying with at the moment?*
- Yeah.

Example 5: Takuma

'I like respite a week you see holiday sure. Shopping and shopping, go shopping lunch on today, Tuesday and Friday. My brother is John Wednesdays and weekends he comes. House in a road. Yeah that's it shopping go shopping and coke. Eh hair get married. He's OK Tony [*Tony is the keyworker*]. Next year. [*Sings*] One day at a time sweet Jesus. Yeah little boy in the pub. [*Puts both thumbs up in the air.*] Perfect – magic.'

Bibliography

Books, articles and manuscripts

Abbott, P. and Sapsford, R., *Community Care for Mentally Handicapped Children*. Milton Keynes: Open University Press 1987.

Alaszewski, A. and Roughton, H., 'The Development of Residential Care for Children with Mental Handicap', in A. Alaszewski and B. N. Ong (eds), *Normalisation in Practice: Residential Care for Children with Profound Mental Handicap*. London: Routledge 1990.

American Association on Mental Deficiency, *Manual on Terminology and Classification in Mental Retardation*. Illinois, Chicago: Herber 1961.

Argyle, M., *Social Encounters: Readings in Social Interaction*. Harmondsworth: Penguin 1978.

Aristotle, *De Anima*, trans. Hugh Lawson-Tancred. Harmondsworth: Penguin 1986.

Aristotle, *The Politics*, revised T. J. Saunders, trans. T. A. Sinclair. Harmondsworth: Penguin 1981.

Ayer, A. J., *The Central Question of Philosophy*. Harmondsworth: Penguin Books 1976.

Baldock, J. and Ungerson, C., *Becoming Consumers of Community Care*. York: Joseph Rowntree Foundation 1994.

Barr, M. and Maloney, E., *1921 Types of Mental Defectives*. London: P. Blakiston 1904.

Barron, D., 'Life in a Mental Institution', in P. Murray and J. Penman (eds), *Telling Our Own Stories: Reflections on Family Life in a Disabling World*. Sheffield: Parents with Attitude 2000.

Bayley, M., *Mental Handicap & Community Care: A Study of Mentally Handicapped People in Sheffield*. London and Boston, MA: Routledge & Kegan Paul 1973.

Bercovici, S., 'Qualitative Methods and Cultural Perspectives in the Study of Deinstitutionalisation', in R. Bruininks, C. Meyers, B. Sigford and K. Lakin (eds), *Deinstitutionalisation and Community Adjustment of Mentally Retarded People*. Monograph, Washington, DC: American Association of Mental Deficiency 1986.

Beresford, P., 'Researching Citizen Involvement: a Collective or Colonizing Enterprise'?, in M. Barnes and G. Wistow (eds), *Researching User Involvement*. London: Nuffield Institute for Health Services Studies 1992.

Beresford, P. and Campbell, J., 'Disabled People, Service Users, Users Involvement and Representation', *Disability and Society* 9, no. 3 (1994): 315–25.

Beresford, P. and Croft, S., *Getting Involved: a Practical Manual*. London: Open Services Project 1993.

Bewley, C. and Glendinning, C., *Involving Disabled People in Community Care Planning*. York: Joseph Rowntree Foundation/Community Care 1994.

Binding, K. and Hoche, A., *The Release of the Destruction of Life Devoid of Life*. Leipzig: F. Meiner 1920.

Bovell, V., Lewis, J. and Wookey, F., 'The Implications for Social Services Departments of the Information Tasks in the Social Care Market', *Health and Social Care in the Community 5*, no. 2 (London 1997).

Brandon, D., *Money for Change*. Cambridge: Anglia Polytechnic University 1994.

Bransbury, L., 'The Right Model for Delivering Social Services?', in L. Bransbury (ed), *The Future of Social Services? Lessons for Best Value from the Purchaser/Provider Split*. London: Local Government Unit (year not given).

Breeching, A. and Walmsley, J. (eds), *Making Connections: Reflecting on the Lives and Experiences of People with Learning Difficulties: A Reader*. Milton Keynes: Open University 1989.

Brown, H., 'Editorial', *Tizard Learning Disability Review* 1, no. 2: 7–8.

Bulmer, H., 'Social Problems as Collective Behaviour', *Social Rights* 18, no. 3: 298–306.

Bulmer, M., *Social Research Ethics* (London: Macmillan 1982); ed. H. Dean as *Ethics and Social Research*, Luton: University of Luton Press and Social Policy Association 1996.

Bulmer, M., *The Social Basis of Community Care*. London: Unwin Hyman 1987.

Campaign for the Mentally Handicapped, *Whose Children?* London: CMH (now Values into Action). 1975.

Campaign for People with Mental Handicaps, *The Principles of Normalisation: A Foundation for Effective Services*. London: CMH, 1981.

Carer's National Association, '*Still Battling?': The Carer's Act One Year on*. London: CNA 1997.

Carkhuff, R. R., *Helping and Human Relations*. New York: Holt 1969.

Centre for Applied Social Studies, University College of Swansea, "User Management in Care Organisations – How users Manage", seminar report. April 1991.

Challis, David and Davies, Bleddyn, *Case Management in Community Care*. Aldershot: Gower 1986.

Clarke, A. M. and Clarke, A. D. B., *Mental Deficiency: The Changing Outlook*, London: Methuen 1958.

Cohen, L. and Manion, L., *Research Methods in Education*, 3rd edn. London: Routledge 1989.

Collins Concise Dictionary of the English Language, 2nd edn, P. Hanks (ed). London/Glasgow: Collins.

Collins, J., *When the Eagles Fly: A Report on Resettlement of People with Learning Difficulties from Long-stay Institutions*. London: Values into Action 1992.

Collins, J., *The Resettlement Game*. London: Values into Action 1993.

Cranefield, Paul F. and Federn, W., "The Begetting of Fools: An Annotated Translation of Paracelsus' DE GENARTIONE STULTORUM" *Bulletin of the History of Medicine* 41 (1967).

Croft, Suzy and Beresford, P., "User Involvement, Citizenship and Social Policy", *Critical Social Policy*, no. 26 (August 1989).

Dalley, G, 'Beliefs and Behaviour: Professionals and the Policy Process', *Journal of Ageing Studies 5*, (1991): 163–80.

Davies, M., *The Essential Social Worker.* Aldershot: Gower/Community Care 1985.

D'Ardenne, P. and Mahtani, A., *Transcultural Counselling in Action.* London: Sage 1989.

Dean, H. (ed.), *Ethics and Social Research.* Luton: University of Luton Press and Social Policy Association, 1996.

Dennett, D., *Elbow Room.* Oxford: Clarendon Press 1984.

Dexter, M. and Harbert, W., *The Home Help Service.* London: Tavistock 1983.

DiMaggio, P. and Powell, W. W., "The Iron Cage Revisited: Institutional Isomorphism and Collective Rationality in Organisational Fields", in Powell, W. W. and P. DiMaggio (eds), *The New Institutionalism in Organisational Analysis.* Chicago: University of Chicago Press 1991.

Donges, G. S., *Policymaking for the Mentally Handicapped.* Gower 1982.

Down, J. L. (1866) 'Classification of Idiots, Clinical Lecture Reports, London Hospital', in Kanner, L. (ed), *The History of the Care and the Study of the Mentally Retarded.* Springfield: Charles C. Thomas 1964.

Dowson, S., *Who Does What?* London: Values Into Action 1990.

Egan, G., *The Skilled Helper: A Systematic Approach to Effective Helping.* Monterey, CA: Brookes/Cole 1986.

Emerson, E., What is Normalisation?', in H. Smith and C. Hatton (eds), *Normalisation: A Reader for the Nineties.* London: Tavistock/Routledge 1992.

Emerson, E. and Hatton, C., 'Residential Provision for People with Intellectual Disabilities in England, Wales and Scotland', *Journal of Applied Research in Intellectual Disabilities* 11, no. 1 (1998): 1–14.

Emerson, Hatton, Felce and Murphy, *see* Foundation for People with Hearing Disabilities.

Farber, B., *Effects of a Seriously Retarded Child on Family Integration*, monograph by the Society for Research in Child Development, 42, no. 2 (1959).

Foucault, M., *Madness and Civilisation: A History of Insanity in the Age of Reason.* London: Tavistock 1967.

Foundation for People with Learning Disabilities, *Learning Disabilities: the Fundamental Facts*, researched and written by Eric Emerson, Chris Hatton, David Felce and Glynis Murphy. London: FPLD 2001.

Fraser, B., 'Communicting with People with a Profound Learning Disability', in O. Russell (ed), *Seminars in the Psychiatry of Learning Disabilities.* London: Gaskell and the Royal College of Psychiatrists 1997.

Fraser, B., 'Communicating with People with Learning Disabilities', in O. Russell (ed), *Seminars in the Psychiatry of Learning Disabilities*, ed. Oliver Russell. London: Gaskell and the Royal College of Psychiatrists 1997.

Fryers, T, 'Impairment, Disability and Handicap: Categories and Classifications', in O. Russell (ed), *Seminars in the Psychiatry of Learning Disabilities.* London: Gaskell and the Royal College of Psychiatrists 1997.

G. Allan Roeher Institute, *The Power to Choose.* North York: G. Allan Roeher Institute 1989.

Galdstone, D., 'The Changing Dynamics of Institutional Care: The Western Counties Idiot Asylum 1864–1914', in D. Wright and A. Digby (eds), *From*

Idiocy to Mental Deficiency: Historical Perspectives on People with Learning Disabilities. London: Routledge 1996.

Galton, F., *Hereditary Genius: An Inquiry into Its Laws and Consequences*. London: Macmillan 1892 (1869).

Galton, F., *Inquiries into Human Faculty and Its Development*. London: Macmillan 1883.

Garcia, E. E. and De Haven, E. D., 'Use of Operant Techniques in the Establishment of and Generalization of Language: a Review and Analysis', *American Journal of Mental Deficiency* 79 (1974): 169–78.

Glaser, B. and Strauss, A., *The Discovery of Grounded Theory: Strategies for Qualitative Research*. New York: Aldine 1967.

Glass, James M., *Life Unworthy of Life: Racial Phobia and Mass Murder in Hitler's Germany*. New York: Basic Books 1997.

Glennerster, Howard and Le Grand, Julian, 'The Development of Quasi Markets', in 'Welfare Provision in the United Kingdom', *International Journal of Health Services* 25, no. 2 (1995).

Glennerster, Howard and Lewis, Jane, *Implementing the New Community Care*. Buckingham: Open University Press 1996.

Glennerster, Howard, Power, Anne and Travers, Tony, 'A New Era for Social Policy: a New Enlightenment or a New Leviathan?', STICERD working paper 39. London: London School of Economics 1989.

Goffman, E., *Asylums: Essays on the Social Situation of Mental Patients and Other Inmates*. Harmondsworth: Penguin 1968.

Goodwin, S., *Community Care and the Future of Mental Health Service Provision: Studies of Care in the Community*, 1st edn. Aldershot: Avebury Gower 1990.

Grant, G. 'Consulting to Involve, or Consulting to Empower', in P. Ramcharan, G. Roberts, G. Grant and J. Borland (eds), *Empowerment in Everyday Life*. London: Jessica Kingsley 1997.

Grey, L. M. and Jenkins, J., 'Investigating Service Satisfaction among People with Learning Difficulties', *Clinical Psychology Forum* 67, (1994): 20–2.

Grisso, T. *Evaluating Competencies: Forensic Assessments and Instruments*. New York: Plenum Press 1986.

Guess, D., Benson, H. A. and Siegel-Causey, E., 'Concept and Issues related to Choice-making and Autonomy among Persons with Severe Disabilities', *Journal of the Association for Severe Handicaps* 10, no. 2 (1985): 79–86.

Gutch, R., *Contracting Lessons from the US*. London: National Council of Voluntary Organisations [NCVO] 1992.

Hanson, D. J., 'Relationship between Methods and Judges in Attitude Behaviour Research', *Psychology* 17, (1980): 11–13, 126, 191.

Harper, G., "Consumer-led Service Planning", *Community Living* 1, no. 6 (1988).

Hillard, L. T. and Kirman, B. H., *Mental Deficiency*. London: Churchill 1957.

Hills, J., *The State of Welfare*. Oxford: Clarendon Press 1990.

Hobbes, T., *Leviathan*, M. Oakeshott (ed). Oxford: Blackwell 1966.

Hobbes, T., *The Elements of Law*, 2nd edn, F. Tonnies (ed), intro. M. M. Goldsmith. London: Simpkin, Marshall 1969.

Holman, A. and Collins, J., *Funding Freedom: Direct Payments for People with Learning Difficulties*. London: Values Into Action 1997.

Hoyes, L. and Harrison, L., 'An Ordinary Private Life', *Community Care*, 12 February 1987: 20–1.

Hudson, B., 'Collaboration in Social Welfare: a Framework for Analysis', *Policy & Politics* 15, no. 3 (1987): 175–82.

Iacono, T., Carter, M. and Hook, J., 'Identification of Intentional Communication in Students with Severe and Multiple Disabilities', *Augmentative and Alternative Communication* 14 (1998): 102–14.

Inman, K., "Testing Times", *Guardian*, 5 April 2000.

Jenkins, J. and Grey, L., 'Multidisciplinary Audit by a Service for People with Learning Disabilities: Quality Assurance and Customers' Views', *Clinical Psychology Forum* 69 (1994): 22–9.

Jones, K., *Asylums & After: a Revised History of the Mental Health Services: from the Early 18th Century to the 1900s*. London: Athlone Press 1993.

Jones, W. T., *A History of Western Philosophy*, Vol. I: *The Classical Mind*, 2nd edn. New York: Harcourt Brace Jovanovich 1970.

Kanner, L., *The History of the Care and Study of the Mentally Retarded*. Springfield, IL: Charles C. Thomas 1964.

Keane, N. and Breo, D, *The Surrogate Mother*. New York: Everest House 1981.

Kelves, D, *In the Name of Eugenics*. Harmondsworth: Penguin 1986.

Kendon, A., 'Some Functions of Gaze-Direction in Social Interaction', in M. Argyle (ed.), *Social Encounters: Readings in Social Interaction*. Harmondsworth: Penguin 1973.

Kiernan, C. and Reid, B., *The Preverbal Communication Schedule (PVCS)*. Windsor: NFER/Nelson 1987.

Knapp, M., Cambridge, P., Thomason, C., Beecham, J., Allen C. and Darton, R., *Care in the Community: Lessons from a Demonstration Programme*. Canterbury: University of Kent, Personal Social Services Research Unit, 1990.

Lart, L. R., Means, R. and Taylor, M., *Community Care in Transition*. York: Joseph Rowntree Foundation 1994.

Le Grand, J. and Bartlett, W., *Quasi Markets in Social Policy*. London: Macmillan 1993.

Lewis, J., 'Purchaser/Provider Splits in Social Care: Context and Issues', in L. Bransbury (ed), *The Future of Social Services? Lessons for Best Value from the Purchaser/Provider Split*. London: Local Government Unit (no year given).

Lishman, J., *Communication in Social Work*. Basingstoke/London: Macmillan 1994.

Lofland, J. and Lofland, L. H., *Analysing Social Settings: a Guide to Qualitative Observation and Analysis*, 2nd edn. Belmont, CA: Wadsworth 1984.

Macintosch, M., 'Flexible Contracting? Economics Cultures and Implicit Contracts in Social Care Partnership'. Buckingham: Open University Press, unpublished paper, 1997.

MacKeith, Caroline, 'A Young Woman's Diary from 1901', in P. Murray and J. Penman (eds), *Telling Our Own Stories: Reflections on Family Life in a Disabling World*. Sheffield: Parents With Attitude 2000.

Malin, N., *Services for People with Learning Disabilities*. London: Routledge 1995.

Malin, N., Race, D. and Jones, G., *Services for the Mentally Handicapped in Britain*. London: Croom Helm 1980.

Mansell, J., 'The Natural History of the Community Mental Handicap Team', in S. Brown and G. Wistow (eds), *The Roles & Tasks of Community Mental Handicap Teams*. Aldershot: Averbury 1990.

Marlet, N. J. and MacLean, H., "A New Lifestyle for Persons With Severe Disabilities: Supported Independence", MS, 1987.

Martin, F. M., *Between the Acts: Community Mental Health Services 1959–1983*. Nuffield Provincial Hospitals Trust, London 1984.

Masland, R. Sarason, S. and Gladwin, T., *Mental Subnormality*. New York: Basic Books 1958.

McGrath, Morag, "Consumer Participation in Service Planning – the AWS Experience", *Journal of Social Policy* 18, part 1 (1989).

McGrath, Morag and Grant, Gordon, "Supporting Needs-Led Services: Implications for Planning and Management", *Journal of Social Policy* 21, part 1 (1992).

McGrath, Morag and Humphreys, S., *The All Wales Community Mental Handicap Team Survey*. Bangor: University College of North Wales 1988.

McIntyre, P., 'Is this the New Genetic Science Eugenics in Disguise?', *Viewpoint*, [The learning disability newspaper from Mencap, London], no. 59. (June/July 2001): 3.

McIver, S., *Obtaining the Views of Users of Health Services*. London: King's Fund 1992.

McKenny, B., "Proposal for Individualized Funding (Draft Three)". Vancouver: Community Living Society 1991.

McKnight, J., "Regenerating Community", address to the Search Conference of the Canadian Mental Health Association, Ottawa, 28 November, 1985.

McLean, L. K. Brady, N. C. and McLean, J. E., 'Reported Communication Abilities of Individuals with Severe Mental Retardation', *American Journal on Mental Retardation* 100 (1996): 580–91. Nuffield Hospital Trust, London.

Means, R. and Smith, R., *Community Care Policy & Practice*. London: Macmilian 1994.

Mencap, *Viewpoint* [the learning disability newspaper] no. 59 (June/July 2001).

Mental Health Foundation, *see* The Mental Health Foundation.

Metro, "On the Threshold of "Immortal Mankind"", 26 June 2000.

Mill, J. S., *An Examination of Sir William Hamilton's Philosophy*. London: Longman 1867.

Mitchell, D. R., 'Parents' Interactions for Mentally Handicapped People', in *Mentally Handicapped People*. M. Beveridge, G. Conti-Ramsden and I. Leudar (eds). London: Chapman & Hall 1987.

Moncrieff, J., *Mental Subnormality in London A Survey of Community Care*, A Political & Economic Planning Report, London, 1966.

Monette, R. D., Sullivan, J. T. and Dejong, R. C., *Applied Social Research Tool for Human Services*. New York: CBS College Publishing 1986.

Moore, C., "Mind the Gap", *Guardian*, 13 March 2002.

Morris, C. D., Niederbuhl, J. N. and Mahr, M., 'Determining the Capability of Individuals with Mental Retardation to give Informed Consent', *American Journal on Mental Retardation* 98, no. 2 (1993): 263–72.

Morris, P., *Put Away: a Sociological Study of Institutions for the Mentally Retarded*. London: Routledge & Kegan Paul 1969.

Morris, J., *Pride Against Prejudice*. London Women's Press 1991.

Munro, E., *Understanding Social Work: An Empirical Approach*. London: Athlone Press 1998.

Murphy, E., *After the Asylums: Community Care for People with Mental Illness.* London: Faber & Faber 1991.

Murphy, J. G., "Incompetence and Paternalism", in his *Retribution, Justice and Therapy.* Dordrecht: Reidel 1979.

Murray, P., 'Personal Reflections on Voice', in *Telling Our Own Stories: Reflections on Family Life in a Disabling World.* P. Murray and J. Penman (eds). Sheffield: Parents with Attitude 2000.

O'Brien, J., *Learning from Citizen Advocacy.* Place, GA: Georgia Citizen Advocacy Office 1987.

O'Brien, J. and Lyle, C., *Introducing Framework for Accomplishment.* Lithonia, GA: Responsive Systems Associates 1986.

Oliver, M., *The Politics of Disablement.* London: Macmillian 1990.

Oliver, M., *Understanding Disability: From Theory to Practice.* London: Macmillan 1996.

O'Neill, O., "Paternalism and Partial Autonomy", *Journal of Medical Ethics*, no. 10 (1984).

Oskamp, S., 'Methods of Studying Social Behaviour', in L. S. Wrightsman, (ed.), *Social Psychology*, 2nd edn. Monterey, CA: Brooks/Cole, 1977.

Oswin, M., 'An Historical Perspective', in C. Robinson and K. Stalker (eds) *Growing up with Disability.* London: Jessica Kingsley 1998.

Peck, E. and Smith, H., *"Safeguarding Service Users"* [Health Service Journal], (7 December 1989).

People First, *Oi! It's My Assessment. Why Not Listen to Me!* London: People First 1993.

Philpot, T. and Ward, L., *Values & Visions: Changing Ideas in Services for People with Learning Difficulties.* Oxford: Butterworth-Heinemann 1995.

Plato, *The Republic*, 2nd edn, trans. Desmond Lee, Harmondsworth: Penguin 1974.

Porter, R., *Mind Forg'd Manacles.* London: Athlone Press 1987.

Powers, J. and Goode, D., 'Enhancing the Quality of Life of Persons with Disabilities Through Incentives Management' unpublished manuscript. New York: Rose F. Kennedy Centre/Albert Einstein College of Medicine 1986.

Prochaska, F., *The Voluntary Impulse: Philanthropy in Modern Britain.* London: Faber & Faber 1988.

Radford, J. P. and Tipper, A., *Starcross: Out of the Mainstream.* Downsview: G. Allan Roeher Institute 1988.

Rawls, J., *A Theory of Justice.* Cambridge, MA: Belknap Press 1971.

Raymond, J. (ed.), *Empowerment in Community Care.* London: Chapman & Hall, 1995.

Rees, R. and Wallace, A., *Verdicts on Social Work.* London: Edward Arnold 1982.

Reith, D., 'I Wonder if You Can Help Me?' *Social Work Today* 6 (1975).

Roberts, G., 'Capacity and Empowerment', in Ramcharan, P., Roberts, G., Grant, G. and Borland, J. (eds) *Empowerment in Everyday Life.* London: Jessica Kingsley 1997.

Robottom, I. and Colquhoun, D., 'The Politics of Method in Public Health Research', in D. Colquhoun and A. Kellehear (eds), *Health Research in Practice: Political, Ethical and Methodological Issues.* London: Chapman & Hall 1993, p. 50.

Robson, C, *Real World Research: A Resource for Social Scientists & Practitioner-Researchers.* MA: Blackwall Publishers 1993.

Rose, S. M. and Black, B. L., *Advocacy and Empowerment*. Boston: Routledge & Kegan Paul 1985.

Rosen, M., Floor, L. and Zisfein, L., 'Investigating the Phenomenon of Acquiescence in the Mentally Handicapped', *Journal of Subnormality* 20 (1974): 58–68.

Salisbury, B., Dickey, J. and Crawford, C., *Service Brokerage: Individual Empowerment and Social Service Accountability*. Downsview: G. Allan Roeher Institute 1987.

Scheerenberger, R. C., *A History of Mental Retardation*. Baltimore, MD: Paul H. Brookes 1983.

Schwartz, W., 'Thoughts from Abroad: Some Perspectives on the Practice of Social Work', *Social Work Today* 14 (1973).

Scull, A., *Museums of Madness: The Social Organisation of Insanity in Nineteenth-Century England*. London: Allen Lane 1979.

Searle, G. R., "Eugenics and Class", in *Biology, Medicine and Society 1840–1940*. Charles Webster (ed). Cambridge: Cambridge University Press 1981.

Seligman, M. E. P., *Helplessness on Depressions, Development, and Death*. San Francisco: Freeman 1975.

Shevin, M. and Klien, N. K., 'The Importance of Choice Making for Students with Severe Disabilities, *Journal of the Association for Severe Disabilities* 9, no. 3 (1984): 159–66.

Shuttleworth, G., *Mentally Deficient Children: Their Treatment and Training*. London: H. K. Lewis 1895.

Simons, K., *I'm Not Complaining, but . . . Complaints Procedures in Social Service Departments*. York: Joseph Rowntree Foundation 1995.

Simons, K., *A Place at the Table? Involving People with Learning Difficulties in Purchasing and Commissioning Services*. Plymouth: British Institute for Learning Difficulties [BILD] 1999.

Smith, D., *Pieces of Purgatory: Mental Retardation in and out of Institutions*. Belmonth, CA: Brooks/Cole, a division of Wadsworth 1995.

Smith, H. and Brown, H, 'Inside Out: a Psychodynamic Approach to Normalisation', in H. Brown and H. Smith (eds) *Normalisation: A Reader for the Nineties*. London and New York: Tavistock/Routledge 1992.

Smith, L., "Lewis", in *Telling Our Own Stories: Reflections on Family Life in a Disabling World*. P. Murray and J. Penman (eds). Sheffield: Parents with Attitude 2000.

Spencer, D., 'Some Implications of the Best Value Regime', in *The Future of Social Services? Lessons for Best Value from the Purchaser/Provider Split*. L. Bransbury (ed). London: Local Government Unit [year not given].

Sperlinger, D. and McAuslane, L., 'Listening to Users of Services for People with Dementia', *Clinical Psychology Forum* 72 (1994): 2–4.

Spradley, J. P., *Participant Observation*. New York: Holt, Rinehart & Winston 1980.

Stainton, T., 'A Terrible Danger to the Race', *Community Living*, 5(3) (January 1992): 18–20.

Stainton, T., *Autonomy & Social Policy: With Special Reference to Mental Handicap in Ontario and Britain*. Aldershot: Ashgate Publishing, 1994; Brookfield, VT: Avebury.

Stalker, K., '*Share the Care': An Evaluation of a Family Based Respite Care Services*. London: Jessica Kingsley 1990.

Sutherland, G. in collaboration with Sharp, Stephen, *Ability, Merit and Measurement: Mental Testing and English Education 1880–1940*. Oxford: Clarendon Press 1984.

Taylor, S. J. and Bogdan, R, 'A Qualitative Approach to the Study of Community Adjustment', in R. H. Bruininiks, C. E. Meyers, B. B. Lakin and K. C. Lakin (eds), *Deinstitutionalisation and Community Adjustment of Mentally Retarded People*, monograph 4. Washington, DC: AAMD 1981.

The Mental Health Foundation, *Building Expectations: Opportunities and Services for People with Learning Disability*. London: MHF 1996.

The Mental Health Foundation, 'Working with People with Severe, Profound and Multiple Learning Difficulties', bulletin 5. London: MHF 1999.

The Mental Health Foundation, *Everyday Lives, Everyday Choices*. London: MHF 2000.

Thomas, S., 'A Meeting in McDonalds', in *Telling Our Own Stories: Reflections on Family Life in a Disabling World*. P. Murray and J. Penman (eds). Sheffield: Parents with Attitude 2000.

Tizard, J. and Grad, J. C., *The Mentally Handicapped and Their Families*. Maudsley Monograph no. 9. London: Maudsley Hospital 1961.

Tizard, J., *Community Services for the Mentally Handicapped*. Oxford: Oxford University Press 1964.

Towell, D., 'An ordinary life: comprehensive locally-based residential services form mentally handicapped', project paper no. 24, reprint. London: King's Fund 1982.

Tredgold, A. F., 'The Feebleminded – a Social Danger', *Eugenics Review* 1 (London 1909): 97–104.

Tredgold, A. F., *A Textbook on Mental Deficiency (Amentia)*. assisted by Tredgold, R. F., London: Bailliére, 1952.

Tuke, D. H., *History of the Insane*. London: Kegan Paul Trench 1882.

Tylor, C., (ed.), *Samuel Tuke (1784–1857): His Life, Work and Thoughts*. London: Headley 1990.

Van der Gaag, A., 'Communication Skills and Adults with Learning Disabilities: Eliminating Professional Myopia', *British Journal of Learning Disabilities* 26 (1998): 88–93.

Van DeVeer, D., *Paternalistic Intervention*. Princeton, NJ: Princeton University Press 1986.

Walker, D., "Paternalism and the Mildly Retarded", *Philosophy and Public Affairs* 8, no. 4 (1979).

Ward, L., "Forward", in *Normalisation: A Reader for the Nineties*, H. Brown and H. Smith (eds). London: Tavistock/Routledge 1992.

Ward, L., 'Equal Citizens: Current Issues for People with Learning Difficulties and Their Allies', in *Values & Visions: Changing Ideas in Services for People with Learning Difficulties*, T. Philpot and L. Ward (eds). Oxford: Butterworth-Heinemann 1995.

Warfield, B. B., "Introductory Essay on Augustine and the Pelagian Controversy", in *A Select Library of the Nicene and Post-Nicene Fathers of the Christian Church*, Vol. 5, *Saint Augustin: Anti-Pelagian Writings*, P. Schaff (ed). Grand Rapids: Wm B. Eerdmans 1956.

Webb, A, 'Co-ordination, a Problem in Public Sector Management', *Policy & Politics*, 19, no. 4 (1991): 29–42.

Whyte, W., Foote, W, *Participatory Action Research*. London: Sage 1991, pp. 20–1.

Wilkener, D., "Paternalism and the Mildly Retarded", *Philosophy and Public Affairs* 8, no. 4 (1979): 391.

Williams, P., 'The Nature and Foundations of the Concept of Normalisation', in Kracas, E. (ed.), *Current Issues in Clinical Psychology* 2. New York: Penguin Press 1985.

Wolfensberger, W., *The Principles of Normalization in Human Services*. Toronto: National Institute on Mental Retardation 1972.

Wolfensberger, W., "A Brief Overview of The Principle of Normalization", in *Normalization, Social Integration and Community Services*, R. J. Flynn and K. E. Nitsch (eds). Baltimore, MD: University Park Press 1980a.

Wolfensberger, W., "The Definition of Normalization: Update, Problems, Disagreements and Misunderstandings", in *Normalization, Social Integration and Community Services*, R. J. Flynn and K. E. Nitsch (eds). Baltimore MD: University Park Press 1980b.

World Health Organisation, *International Classification of Impairments, Disabilities and Handicaps*. Geneva: WHO 1980.

Worrell, B., *Advice For Advisors*. Downsview: National People First Project 1988.

Public documents, reports and publications

Audit Commission, *Making a Reality of Community Care*. London: HMSO 1986.

Bone, M. and Meltzer, H., *The Prevalence of Disability Among Children*. report no. 3. London: OPCS, HMSO 1989.

Department of Environment, Transport and the Regions, *Modernising Local Government: Improving Local Services through Best Value*. London: HMSO 1998.

Department of Health, *Mental Health Act (Part 1 Section 4)*. London: HMSO 1959.

Department of Health, *Disabled Persons (Services, Consultation & Representation) Act*. London: HMSO 1986.

Department of Health, *Caring for People: Community Care in the Next Decade and Beyond*. London: HMSO 1989a.

Department of Health, *Modernising Social Services, Promoting Independence, Improving Protection, Raising Standards*. Cm. 4169. London: HMSO 1989b.

Department of Health, *Implementing Community Care: Purchaser, Commissioner and Provider Roles*. London: HMSO 1991.

Department of Health, *The Carers (Recognition and Services) Act*. London: HMSO 1995.

Department of Health, *Direct Payment Act: Policy & Practice*. London: HMSO 1996.

Department of Health, *NHS Act*. London: HMSO 1977.

Department of Health, *Partnership in Action (New Opportunities for Joint Working between Health and Social Services*', a discussion document. London: HMSO 1998.

Department of Health, *Caring About Carers: A National Strategy for Carers*. London: HMSO 1999.

Department of Health, *Guidance on the Health Act Section 31 Partnership Arrangements*. London: HMSO 1999.

Department of Health, *Valuing People: A New Strategy for Learning Disability for the 21st Century.* a White Paper, Cm 5086. London: HMSO 2001.

Department of Health, *Valuing People: A New Strategy for Learning Disability for the 21st Century: Implementation.* Implementation Guidance, Health Service Circular Local Authority Circular, Series Number: LAC(2001)23. London: HMSO 2002.

Department of Health & Social Security, *Better Services for the Mentally Handicapped.* London: HMSO 1971.

Department of Health and Social Services Inspectorate, *Purchase of Services Guidance.* London: HMSO 1991.

Griffiths, Sir R., *Community Care: Agenda for Action.* a Report to the Secretary of State for Social Services. London: HMSO 1988.

Howe Report, *Report of the Committee of Inquiry into Allegations of Ill Treatment of Patients and Other Regularities at the Ely Hospital, Cardiff.* Cmnd 3975. London: HMSO 1969.

Jay Report, *Committee of Inquiry into Mental Handicap Nursing & Care*, Vol. 1. Cmnd 7468–1. London: HMSO 1979.

Law Commission, *Mental Incapacity.* London: HMSO 1995.

Lord Chancellor's Department, *Who Decided? Making Decisions on Behalf of Mentally Incapacitated Adults.* London: The Stationery Office 1997.

Mental Deficiency 1954–1957, *Report and Minutes of Evidence.* Cmnd 169. London: HMSO 1957.

National Council for Civil Liberties, *50,000 Outside the Law.* London: NCCL 1951.

Registrar-General, *Statistical Review of England & Wales* (1960), *Supplement on Mental Health, Report of the Committee on Local Authority Personal Social Services* (The Seebohm Report). Home Office Department of Education & Science, Ministry of Health, 1968. Cmnd 3703. London: HMSO.

Royal Commission on the Care and Control of the Feeble-Minded, *Minutes of Evidence*, Vols. I-VII, *Report*, Vol. VIII. Parliamentary Papers, Vols. XXXV-XXXIX. 1908.

Royal Commission on the Law Relating to Mental Illness & Mental Deficiency, 1954–1957, *Minutes of Evidence.* London: HMSO 1957.

Social Services Committee, *Second Report: Community Care.* House of Commons Paper 13–1, Sessions 1984–5. London: HMSO 1985.

Social Services Inspectorate, *Care Management and Assessment: Manager's Guide.* London: HMSO 1991.

Social Services Inspectorate, *Opportunity or Knocks: National Inspection of Recreation and Leisure in Day Services for People with Learning Difficulties.* London: DOH 1995.

The Idiots Act, Parliamentary Papers, Vol. II. 1886.

Wagner, G., *Residential Care: A Positive Choice.* Report of the Independent Review of Residential Care, National Institute for Social Work. London: HMSO 1988.

Watkins Report, *Report of the Farleigh Hospital Committee of Inquiry.* Cmnd 4557. London: HMSO 1971.

Western Counties Asylums Annual Report. Exeter: Northcott Devon Medical Foundation 1902.

Internet references

"Eugenics": http://www.encarta.msm.com/find/concise
"Existentialism": this is the Existentialism page: http://www.connect.net
"Getting Control of the Money": http://www.viauk.org
Guidance on the Health Act Section 31 Partnership Arrangements. London, Department of Health Publications on the Internet: http://www.doh.gov.uk
"Handicapped" published by the United States Holocaust Memorial Museum: http://www.ushmm.org
"Let them Speak" (17–9–2000): http://www.community-care.co.uk
'Local concerns for learning difficulty white paper aims' (3–5–2001): http://www.community-are.co.uk
London Learning Disability Strategy Reference Group: DOH, SSI and NHS: http://www.doh.gov.uk
"Paracelsus" http://www.nlm.nih.gov.uk
"Philippe Pinel"- encyclopaedia article from Britannica.com: http://www.britannica.com/seo/p/philippe-pinel/
Quaker Views – Introduction: Making Decisions' and 'A Glossary of Quaker Terms': http://www.quaker.org.uk/more/qviews/qviews1.html
"Sartre, Jean-Paul": http://www.encarta.msn.com
"The Final Struggle and the Victory of Science–Pinel and Tuke": http://www.santafe.edu
"What is Learning Disability?": http://www.mencap.org.uk
"Will" (Philosophy and Psychology): http://www.encarta.msn.com

Resource centres and technology centres

AbilityNet SouthEast, c/o IBM United Kingdom, Unit 9, Weybridge Business Park, Addlestone Road, Weybridge Surrey KT15 2UK. Tel: 01932 814558. Fax: 01932 814559. e-mail: sue@abilitynet.org.uk (AbilityNet SouthEast is a charity formed to help people with disabilities gain easier access to computer technology.)
British Institute for Learning Disabilities, Wolverhampton Road, Kidderminster, Worcester DY0 3PP. Tel: 01562 850251. Fax: 01562 851970. e-mail: bild@bild.demon.co.uk
Central England People First Limited, P.O. Box 5200, Northampton NN1 1ZB. Tel: 01604 721 666. Fax: 01604 721 6111. e-mail: northants@peoplefirst.org.uk
Mencap, 123 Golden Lane, London EC1Y 0RT. Tel: 020 7454 0454. Fax: 020 7696 5540. e-mail: information@mencap.org.uk
Norah Fry Research Centre, University of Bristol, 3 Priory Road, Bristol BS8 1TX. Tel: 0117 923 8132. Fax: 0117 946 6553.
Paradigm, 24 Brancote Road, Oxton, Wirral CH43 6TJ. Tel: 0151 652 4484. Fax: 0151 651 0183. e-mail: admin@paradigm-uk.demon.co.uk
Pavillion Publishing, The Ironworks, Cheapside, Brighton, East Sussex BN1 46D. Tel: 1273 623 222. Fax: 1273 625 526. e-mail: info@parpub.com
The Foundation for People with Learning Disabilities, UK Office, 7th Floor, 83 Victoria Street, London SW1H 0HW. Tel: 020 7802 0300. Fax: 020 7802 0301. e-mail: fpld@fpld.org.uk

The Mental Health Foundation, UK Office, 7th Floor, 83 Victoria Street, London SW1H 0HW. Tel: 020 7802 0300. Fax: 020 7802 0301. e-mail: mhf@mhf.org.uk

The National Autistic Society, 393 City Road, London EC1V 1NG. Tel: 020 7833 2299. Fax: 020 7833 9666. e-mail: nas@nas.org.uk

Tizard Centre, University of Kent at Canterbury, Canterbury, Kent CT2 7LZ. Tel: 01227 764000. Fax: 01227 763674. e-mail: tizardgen@ukc.ac.uk

Values Into Action, Oxford House, Derbyshire Street, London E2 6HG. Tel: 020 7729 5436. Fax: 020 7729 7792. e-mail: general@viauk.org.uk

List of tables

List of figures

Index